Current Topics in Anesthesia for Head and Neck Surgery

Guest Editors

JOSHUA H. ATKINS, MD, PhD
JEFF E. MANDEL, MD

ANESTHESIOLOGY CLINICS

www.anesthesiology.theclinics.com

Consulting Editor
LEE A. FLEISHER, MD, FACC

September 2010 • Volume 28 • Number 3

SAUNDERS an imprint of ELSEVIER, Inc.

W.B. SAUNDERS COMPANY
A Division of Elsevier Inc.

1600 John F. Kennedy Boulevard, Suite 1800 • Philadelphia, PA 19103-2899
http://www.theclinics.com

ANESTHESIOLOGY CLINICS Volume 28, Number 3
September 2010 ISSN 1932-2275, ISBN-13: 978-1-4377-2425-7

Editor: Rachel Glover
Developmental Editor: Donald Mumford

Anesthesiology Clinics (ISSN 1932-2275) is published quarterly by Elsevier Inc., 360 Park Avenue South, New York, NY 10010-1710. Months of issue are March, June, September, and December. Periodicals postage paid at New York, NY and at additional mailing offices. Subscription prices are $134.00 per year (US student/resident), $268.00 per year (US individuals), $328.00 per year (Canadian individuals), $417.00 per year (US institutions), $517.00 per year (Canadian institutions), $189.00 per year (Canadian and foreign student/resident), $372.00 per year (foreign individuals), and $517.00 per year (foreign institutions). To receive student and resident rate, orders must be accompanied by name of affiliated institution, date of term, and the *signature* of program/residency coordinator on institutions letterhead. Orders will be billed at individual rate until proof of status is received. Foreign air speed delivery is included in all *Clinics'* subscription prices. All prices are subject to change without notice. POSTMASTER: Send address changes to *Anesthesiology Clinics,* Elsevier Health Sciences Division, Subscription Customer Service, 3251 Riverport Lane, Maryland Heights, MO 63043. Customer Service (orders, claims, online, change of address): Elsevier Health Sciences Division, Subscription Customer Service, 3251 Riverport Lane, Maryland Heights, MO 63043. Tel:1-800-654-2452 (U.S. and Canada); 314-447-8871 (outside U.S. and Canada). Fax: 314-447-8029. E-mail: journalscustomerservice-usa@elsevier.com (for print support); journalsonlinesupport-usa@elsevier.com (for online support).

Reprints. For copies of 100 or more of articles in this publication, please contact the Commercial Reprints Department, Elsevier Inc., 360 Park Avenue South, New York, NY 10010-1710. Tel.: 212-633-3812; Fax: 212-462-1935; E-mail: reprints@elsevier.com.

Anesthesiology Clinics, is also published in Spanish by McGraw-Hill Inter-americana Editores S. A., P.O. Box 5-237, 06500 Mexico D. F., Mexico.

Anesthesiology Clinics, is covered in *MEDLINE/PubMed (Index Medicus), Current Contents/Clinical Medicine, Excerpta Medica, ISI/BIOMED,* and *Chemical Abstracts.*

Printed and bound by CPI Group (UK) Ltd, Croydon, CR0 4YY

Transferred to Digital Print 2011

Contributors

CONSULTING EDITOR

LEE A. FLEISHER, MD, FACC
Robert D. Dripps Professor and Chair of Anesthesiology and Critical Care, University of Pennsylvania School of Medicine, Philadelphia, Pennsylvania

GUEST EDITORS

JOSHUA H. ATKINS, MD, PhD
Assistant Professor, Department Anesthesiology and Critical Care, University of Pennsylvania, Philadelphia, Pennsylvania

JEFF E. MANDEL, MD, MS
Assistant Professor, Department of Anesthesiology and Critical Care, University of Pennsylvania School of Medicine, Philadelphia, Pennsylvania

AUTHORS

MARTHA R. CORDOBA AMOROCHO, MD
Anesthesiologist, Department of Anesthesiology and Critical Care, Brigham and Women's Hospital, Boston, Massachusetts

JOSHUA H. ATKINS, MD, PhD
Assistant Professor, Department Anesthesiology and Critical Care, University of Pennsylvania, Philadelphia, Pennsylvania

PETER BIRO, MD, DESA
Department of Anesthesiology, Institute of Anesthesiology, University Hospital Zurich, Zurich, Switzerland

JOHN J. CHI, MD
Clinical Assistant Instructor, Department of Otorhinolaryngology–Head and Neck Surgery, University of Pennsylvania School of Medicine, Philadelphia, Pennsylvania

COREY E. COLLINS, DO, FAAP
Director, Pediatric Anesthesia, Department of Anesthesiology, Massachusetts Eye and Ear Infirmary; Instructor, Harvard Medical School, Boston, Massachusetts

FRANCIS X. DILLON, MD
Assistant Anesthetist, Department of Anesthesia, Massachusetts Eye and Ear Infirmary; Instructor, Harvard Medical School, Boston, Massachusetts

PETER R. EASTWOOD, PhD
Professor, West Australian Sleep Disorders Research Institute, Department of Pulmonary Physiology, Sir Charles Gairdner Hospital, Nedlands; School of Anatomy and Human Biology, University of Western Australia, Perth, Western Australia, Australia

JAMES S. GREEN, MBBS, FRCA
Fellow, Department of Anesthesiology and Pain Medicine, University of Alberta, Edmonton, Alberta, Canada

DAVID R. HILLMAN, MD
Professor, West Australian Sleep Disorders Research Institute, Department of Pulmonary Physiology; Department of Anaesthesia, Sir Charles Gairdner Hospital, Nedlands, Perth, Western Australia, Australia

MICHAEL G. IRWIN, MB, ChB, MD, FRCA
Professor and Head, Department of Anaesthesiology, University of Hong Kong, Queen Mary Hospital, Pokfulam, Hong Kong

DEYA N. JOURDY, MD
Department of Otorhinolaryngology, Weill Cornell Medical College, New York, New York

ASHUTOSH KACKER, MD
Associate Professor, Department of Otorhinolaryngology, Weill Cornell Medical College, New York, New York

SHARON LIANG, BSc, MBBS
Medical Officer, Department of Anaesthesiology, Queen Mary Hospital, Pokfulam, Hong Kong

ROBERT G. LOEB, MD
Associate Professor, Clinical Anesthesiology, Department of Anesthesiology, University of Arizona College of Medicine, Tucson, Arizona

JEFF E. MANDEL, MD, MS
Assistant Professor, Department of Anesthesiology and Critical Care, University of Pennsylvania School of Medicine, Philadelphia, Pennsylvania

NATASHA MIRZA, MD
Professor, Department of Otorhinolaryngology, Head and Neck Surgery; Director, Penn Center for Voice and Swallowing, University of Pennsylvania, Philadelphia, Pennsylvania

BERT W. O'MALLEY Jr, MD
Professor and Chairman, Department of Otorhinolaryngology–Head and Neck Surgery, University of Pennsylvania School of Medicine, Philadelphia, Pennsylvania

PETER R. PLATT, MD
Professor, Department of Anaesthesia, Sir Charles Gairdner Hospital, Nedlands, Perth, Western Australia, Australia

DAVID S. SHEINBEIN, MD
Assistant Professor of Anesthesiology, Department of Anesthesiology, University of Arizona College of Medicine, Tucson, Arizona

ANTHONY SORDILLO, DDS, DMD
Associate Anesthesiologist, Massachusetts Eye and Ear Infirmary, Boston, Massachusetts

BAN C.H. TSUI, MD, FRCPC
Professor and Vice Chair (Research), Department of Anesthesiology and Pain Medicine; Director, Regional Anesthesia and Acute Pain Service, University of Alberta, Edmonton, Alberta, Canada

GREGORY S. WEINSTEIN, MD
Professor and Vice Chairman, Department of Otorhinolaryngology–Head and Neck Surgery, University of Pennsylvania School of Medicine, Philadelphia, Pennsylvania

PENG XIAO, MD
Department of Anesthesiology, Massachusetts Eye and Ear Infirmary; Instructor, Harvard Medical School, Boston, Massachusetts

XIANGWEI (SHANNON) ZHANG, MD, MS
Department of Anesthesiology, Massachusetts Eye and Ear Infirmary; Instructor, Harvard Medical School, Boston, Massachusetts

Contents

> The clinical applications of jet ventilation (JV) in ear, nose, and throat surgery can be best understood by the characteristics that distinguish this form of ventilation from conventional positive pressure ventilation. By definition, JV is based on the application of gas portions under high pressure through an unblocked catheter into the airway, which is open to the ambient air. Beneficial opportunities arise in JV, which otherwise are not available in regular ventilation.

> During the past decade, robotic surgery has been progressively incorporated into the mainstream of cardio-thoracic and abdominopelvic surgery. With the recent US Food and Drug Administration approval of transoral robotic surgery (TORS) for the treatment of all benign tumors and select malignant tumors of the head and neck, robotic surgery has established its place in otolaryngologic surgery. Given the multispecialty applications and widespread use of robotic surgery, there exists a need for anesthesiologists to familiarize themselves with robotic surgery. This article focuses on TORS and the goal of which is to provide the anesthesiologist with a foundation for caring for the TORS patient in the perioperative period.

> Intraoperative neuromonitoring (IONM) is a relatively recent advance in electromyography (EMG) applied to otolaryngology-head and neck surgery. Its purpose is to allow real-time identification and functional assessment of vulnerable nerves during surgery. The nerves most often monitored in head and neck surgery are the motor branch of the facial nerve (VII), the recurrent or inferior laryngeal nerves (X), the vagus nerve (X), and the spinal accessory nerve (XI), with other cranial lower nerves monitored less frequently. Morbidity from trauma to these nerves is significant and obvious, such as unilateral facial paresis. Although functional restorative surgery is usually considered to repair the effects of such an insult, the importance of preventing nerve injury in head and neck surgery

is obvious. This article focuses on the anesthetic considerations pertinent to IONM of peripheral cranial nerves during otolaryngologic-head and neck surgery. The specific modality of IONM is EMG, both spontaneous and evoked.

Anesthesia, Sleep, and Upper Airway Collapsibility

David R. Hillman, Peter R. Platt, and Peter R. Eastwood

Anesthesia and sleep both predispose to upper airway obstruction through state-induced reductions in pharyngeal dilator muscle activation and lung volume. The tendencies are related in patients with obstructive sleep apnea commonly presenting with difficulties in airway management in the perioperative period. This is a period of great potential vulnerability for such patients because of compromise of the arousal responses that protect against asphyxiation during natural sleep. Careful preoperative evaluation and insightful perioperative observation are likely to identify patients at risk. A significant proportion of patients will have previously undiagnosed obstructive sleep apnea and anesthesiologists are well placed to identify this potential. Patients with known or suspected obstructive sleep apnea need careful postoperative management, particularly while consciousness and arousal responses are impaired. Specific follow-up of suspected cases is needed to ensure that the sleep-related component of the problem receives appropriate care.

Regional Anesthesia for Office-based Procedures in Otorhinolaryngology

Deya N. Jourdy and Ashutosh Kacker

Local and topical anesthetic techniques have long been used for office-based procedures in otorhinolaryngology. There are numerous advantages to using local and topical anesthesia for office-based procedures, including a shorter recovery period, decreased health care cost, and the maintenance of a conscious patient who can communicate with the surgeon and maintain his or her own airway during the procedure. In this manuscript, we review the local and topical anesthetic techniques that can be used for otorhinolaryngic procedures including anesthesia of the external face, ear, nose, oral cavity, nasopharynx, oropharynx, hypopharynx, and larynx.

Laryngeal Mask Airways in Ear, Nose, and Throat Procedures

Jeff E. Mandel

The use of laryngeal mask airway (LMA) and its variants in ear, nose, and throat procedures have been extensively described in case reports, retrospective reviews, and randomized clinical trials. The LMA has developed a considerable following because of its lack of tracheal stimulation, which can be a considerable advantage in ear, nose, and throat (ENT) procedures. The incidence of coughing on emergence has been shown to be lower with the LMA than with the endotracheal tube (ETT). Although other approaches to smooth emergence have been described, few would argue that it is as easy to achieve a smooth emergence with an ETT as with an LMA. Although patients certainly exist for whom the LMA is contraindicated, many will experience better results with the LMA because of the features delineated in this article.

lesions and malignant lesions. Most benign lesions are treatable with surgery and speech therapy, whereas the malignant lesions require more invasive surgery as well as radiation and chemotherapy. Preoperative assessment and anesthesia management for adult laryngotracheal surgery are reviewed.

This article presents a comprehensive narrative review of the published literature relating to ultrasound imaging relevant to anesthesia for ear, nose, and throat (ENT) surgery. The review comprises 2 main subject areas: the use of ultrasonography related to assessment and management of the airway, and the use of ultrasonography related to nerve blockade for ENT surgery. The relevant sonoanatomy and suitable probe placement are illustrated in relation to applicable regional anatomy (they are not discussed). The possible value of the use of ultrasonography to improve existing clinical practice in these areas is explored.

The evolution of novel techniques for the treatment of laryngeal pathology has led to a significant expansion of the role of diagnostic assessment and the range of laryngeal procedures performed. These procedures typically benefit from an anesthetic approach that diverges from a standard general endotracheal or laryngeal mask airway—based inhalational anesthetic. The shared airway, need for intraoperative assessment of vocal cord function, risk of airway fire, and desire for rapid emergence and discharge are all important factors. In this article the authors undertake a collaborative anesthesia-surgical discussion of anesthetic management for airway procedures that are optimally performed with a spontaneously breathing, cooperative patient. An overview of pharmacologic approaches to airway anesthesia and cooperative sedation, followed by a discussion on the surgical requirements and anesthetic goals of commonly performed procedures, are presented.

FORTHCOMING ISSUES

December 2010
Perioperative Pharmacotherapy
Alan Kaye, MD, *Guest Editor*

March 2011
Quality in Anesthesia
Elizabeth A. Martinez, MD, and
Mark Neuman, MD, *Guest Editors*

June 2011
**Regional Analgesia and Acute Pain
Management**
Sugantha Ganapathy, MD, and
Vincent Chan, MD, *Guest Editors*

RECENT ISSUES

June 2010
Ambulatory Anesthesia
Peter S.A. Glass, MB, ChB,
Guest Editor

March 2010
**Anesthesia for Patients Too Sick
for Anesthesia**
Benjamin A. Kohl, MD, and
Stanley H. Rosenbaum, MD,
Guest Editors

December 2009
**Preoperative Medical Consultation:
A Multidisciplinary Approach**
Lee A. Fleisher, MD, FACC, and
Stanley H. Rosenbaum, MD,
Guest Editors

RELATED INTEREST

Otolaryngologic Clinics of North America April 2010 (Volume 43, Issue 2)
Thyroid and Parathyroid Surgery
Ralph P. Tufano, MD and Sara I. Pai, MD, PhD, *Guest Editors*

THE CLINICS ARE NOW AVAILABLE ONLINE!

Access your subscription at:
www.theclinics.com

Foreword

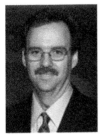

Lee A. Fleisher, MD
Consulting Editor

Anesthesia for head and neck surgery has traditionally not been considered one of the more specialized areas within the field; however, many advances in both surgical techniques as well as airway management and newer drugs have led to advances in care for these patients over the past decade. In particular, minimally invasive surgery has allowed for excision for more invasive tumors with less distortion of the anatomy. New airway devices and techniques have also led to changes in anesthetic management. Finally, short-acting agents have led to the development of techniques which in many cases are safer and allow spontaneous ventilation or easier control of the airway. For these reasons, it became clear that an issue of *Anesthesiology Clinics* devoted to this topic was warranted.

In choosing editors for this issue, I identified faculty from my department at the University of Pennsylvania who have been active in advancing the field. Joshua Atkins, MD, PhD and Jeff Mandel, MD, MS are both currently Assistant Professors of Anesthesiology and Critical Care at the University of Pennsylvania School of Medicine. Josh received his Medical Degree and his PhD in Chemistry from Columbia University and, after his residency at Penn, has been actively involved in anesthesia for head and neck surgery. His research interests have focused on monitoring ventilation and provision of novel sedative regimens. Jeff received his Medical Degree from the University of Texas Health Science Center and a Masters Degree in Engineering and Systems Science from the University of California San Diego. He has a longstanding interest in technology and has been an active member of the Society for Technology in Anesthesia. His recent research interests focus on developing novel target control sedative regimens for patients undergoing procedures such as endoscopy. Together they have invited an impressive list of anesthesiologists and surgeons to update the community on this exciting area of growth.

Lee A. Fleisher, MD
University of Pennsylvania School of Medicine
3400 Spruce Street, Dulles 680
Philadelphia, PA 19104, USA

E-mail address:
fleishel@uphs.upenn.edu

Anesthesiology Clin 28 (2010) xiii
doi:10.1016/j.anclin.2010.08.001
1932-2275/10/$ – see front matter **anesthesiology.theclinics.com**

Preface

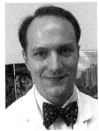 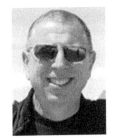

Joshua H. Atkins, MD, PhD   Jeff E. Mandel, MD, MS
Guest Editors

Few would disagree with the notion that anesthesia for head and neck surgery is a significant component of the bread and butter services provided by many anesthesia groups. We surmise that the volume of debate would grow louder if one advocated for the creation of a subspeciality ENT track in training programs and departments. Why should this be?

This issue of the *Anesthesiology Clinics* illustrates that the advent of new technologies such as surgical robots, the increasing expectations of surgeons and patients alike for rapid, asymptomatic recovery, and the extension of established equipment such as ultrasound and LMAs to novel ENT applications would lead many to conclude that head and neck anesthesia is awash with activity. Those who practice ENT anesthesia regularly recognize that the anesthetic model has evolved from a simplistic approach of getting the patient intubated and through the surgery to the broader goals of enhancing OR throughput, emphasizing patient satisfaction, and optimizing operating conditions with subtle anesthetic modifications.

For example, increasingly sophisticated airway procedures for diagnosis and treatment of contained pharyngeal and laryngeal lesions are considered for performance in outpatient settings with mild sedation and topicalization. Newer pharmacologic agents such as dexmedetomidine and remifentanil are gaining traction in the management of sedation for airway surgery. As Atkins and Mirza discuss, these agents are being combined in unique ways with traditional agents such as lidocaine and ketamine to meet anesthetic goals for procedures including medialization thyroplasty and collagen vocal cord injection. This is complemented by Kacker's in-depth discussion of approaches to regional blockade of the ear, nose, oropharynx, and larynx for otorhinologic procedures in the office. Tsui expands on these discussions in an article devoted to the broad applicability of ultrasound to ENT anesthesia.

Evolving strategies to perform procedures in ambulatory surgery centers or surgeon offices are confronted with the challenge of an increasing number of patients with morbid obesity, obstructive sleep apnea, or laryngotracheal pathology. As such, it has become ever more important for the anesthesiologist to understand the functional physiology of airway obstruction and gain mastery of the pharmacology of sedative-hypnotic agents and opioids as it relates to respiratory control. Hillman and colleagues explore in-depth current knowledge in this area.

Anesthesiology Clin 28 (2010) xv–xvi
doi:10.1016/j.anclin.2010.08.002
1932-2275/10/$ – see front matter

The laryngeal mask airway has rapidly evolved from a clinical curiosity to a mainstay device for a great variety of procedures performed under general anesthesia. Traditionally held beliefs such as avoidance of LMAs in patients with GERD, in nonsupine surgical position, and during positive pressure ventilation have gradually eroded. As Mandel illustrates, the use of classic and alternative LMA constructs such as the flexible LMA has become more commonplace and the extension of this practice to a variety of ENT procedures continues. Indeed there may even be distinct advantages to the LMA over endotracheal intubation in selected patients.

The use of total intravenous anesthesia (TIVA) for ENT anesthesia continues to expand. Indeed, the anesthesia community is now being drawn into debate regarding the overall benefits and risks of inhalational versus intravenous anesthesia in the context of patient outcomes. As several authors illustrate, TIVA may be advantageous for properties relating to intraoperative blood pressure, decreased emergence phenomena, and postoperative recovery profile. Surgeons are increasingly inclined to express a preference for anesthetic technique in this regard.

The advance of technology in head and neck surgery continues unabated and with it comes exciting opportunities to adapt anesthetic approaches to novel circumstances. Transoral robotic surgery for tonsillectomy, base of tongue resection, thyroidectomy, and laryngeal cancer treatment is a growing area. The operating room setup, patient positioning, and intraoperative maneuvers are relatively unique and introduced by Chi and Mandel in this issue.

Old technologies such as jet ventilation have seen a resurgence for procedures such as microdirect laryngoscopy and tracheal resection. The advent of automated jet ventilators such as the Acutronic Monsoon with pressure alarms and humidification capability has made routine use of jet ventilation safer and easier than in the past. Biro provides an excellent review of the principles and current state of the art in jet ventilation for airway surgery.

Of course, classic head and neck surgery has not disappeared. Current management strategies for core procedures including laryngeal surgery for cancer patients, pediatric airway surgery, endoscopic sinus surgery, and inner ear surgery are each reviewed. However, ENT surgery is no longer "just another neck" or a "simple tonsil." There are exciting opportunities for progress in anesthesia for head and neck surgery and someday it might not seem embarrassing to call yourself an ENT specialist.

Joshua H. Atkins, MD, PhD
Department of Anesthesiology and Critical Care
University of Pennsylvania
680 Dulles Building
3400 Spruce Street
Philadelphia, PA 19104, USA

Jeff E. Mandel, MD, MS
Department of Anesthesiology and Critical Care
University of Pennsylvania School of Medicine
3400 Spruce Street
Philadelphia, PA 19104, USA

E-mail addresses:
atkinsj@uphs.upenn.edu (J.H. Atkins)
mandelj@uphs.upenn.edu (J.E. Mandel)

Jet Ventilation for Surgical Interventions in the Upper Airway

Peter Biro, MD, DESA

KEYWORDS

- High-frequency jet ventilation • Upper airway surgery
- Microlaryngoscopy • Equipment • Monitoring

The clinical applications of jet ventilation (JV) in ear, nose, and throat surgery can be best understood by the characteristics that distinguish this form of ventilation from conventional positive pressure ventilation. By definition, JV is based on the application of gas portions under high pressure through an unblocked catheter into the airway, which is open to the ambient air.[1] This implies a ventilation system, in which a gas-tight separation of the respiratory system from the environment does not exist. The insufflation of gas through the jet nozzle is an active process whereas the exhalation happens outside the jet nozzle and is passive. This untight coupling of the ventilation system with the airway is unusual for the user, and the same is true when handbag ventilation is not possible. Nevertheless, controlled ventilation is possible as is spontaneous breathing. Another characteristic feature of JV is that the resulting chest movements do not reflect the exchanged gas volumes. For this reason the term, *tidal volume (TV)*, for one JV cycle is not appropriate, because a part of the gas exchange (but not all of it) happens with a smaller expansion of the lungs and the thorax than the administered TV.

Because of these specific features, beneficial opportunities arise in JV, which otherwise are not available in regular ventilation, such as absence of an endotracheal tube (ETT) and unhindered access to the airway by a surgeon. Additionally, surgical instruments and manipulations have less influence or even risks for interfering with the airway maintenance instruments of the anesthetist. These circumstances allow the specific indications of JV for microlaryngoscopic laryngeal surgery, interventional rigid bronchoscopy, or similar interventions.

Institute of Anesthesiology, University Hospital Zurich, Raemistrasse 100, CH-8091 Zurich, Switzerland
E-mail address: peter.biro@usz.ch

Anesthesiology Clin 28 (2010) 397–409
doi:10.1016/j.anclin.2010.07.001   **anesthesiology.theclinics.com**

INDICATIONS

High-frequency JV is useful in all situations where access to the airway by a surgeon is hindered by the anesthesiologic equipment, in particular by an ETT. Conversely, JV is also a favorable ventilation technique if the anesthesiologic equipment might be negatively affected (kinked, obstructed, displaced, damaged, or ignited) by the surgeon. Therefore, JV is used in a way that either does not require an ETT at all or requires only a narrow catheter with resistance to laser beams. Rigid bronchoscopy is another procedure that might benefit from JV; maintenance of gas exchange is easy with JV where a large part of the insufflated gas is lost due to the untight sealing of the airway around the rigid instrument. Even though jet gas immediately flows out to the atmosphere, sufficient ventilation is still possible. This is even more the case if the rigid bronchoscope is used as a pathway for additional instruments, such as rigid optics, microsurgical instruments, and endobronchial ultrasound probes. Under JV, the proximal end of the bronchoscope may be left open, unlike in conventional ventilation, thus facilitating the use of these instruments considerably. The relatively easy and less-invasive transtracheal puncture with a narrow cannula suggest JV as a good indication for emergency oxygenation in a cannot intubate–cannot ventilate scenario. And, finally, the omission of airtight coupling between the jet nozzle and the airway allows the unique opportunity to maintain ventilation even if the airway is disrupted. This is the case in subglottic and tracheal surgery, where the airway might be partially or even totally open to the atmosphere.

There is no absolute contraindication to JV; however, difficulties can be encountered in maintaining oxygenation and/or CO_2 elimination in certain patients. This is the case in morbid obesity, stiff thorax, and, most commonly, advanced forms of restrictive and/or obstructive pneumopathy. Other situations precluding a smooth and successful application of JV are lung fibrosis and reduced alveolar-capillary diffusion capacity, such as in pulmonary edema. All of these can be considered contraindications for JV when a patient's parameters for gas exchange cannot be kept within tolerable limits during JV.

INTERFACES BETWEEN VENTILATOR AND PATIENT

There are three commonly used variants of the jet nozzles position in relation to the airway: infraglottic, supraglottic, and transtracheal JV.

Infraglottic Jet Ventilation

An infraglottic JV configuration is when the jet nozzle is located below the vocal cord level in the trachea.[2] This is the standard version for JV in laryngeal surgery but is also the case when JV is applied via a rigid bronchoscope. Usually a thin jet catheter (1.5–2 mm inner diameter [ID]) is introduced into the airway and positioned with its tip in mid-trachea. Nowadays, a double-lumen LaserJet jet catheter (Acutronic MS, Hirzel, Switzerland) is available, which has an outer diameter of 4.0 mm and is made of incombustible tetrafluorethylene (Teflon). This catheter is usually introduced in the same manner as ETTs, by direct laryngoscopy. This approach has several advantages. First, the airway is secured regardless of a surgeon's actions and equipment; in particular, ventilation can be installed before the suspension laryngoscope is in place and also can be maintained after this device has been removed (**Fig. 1**). This means that JV can be applied from the beginning to the end of anesthesia, without the need to occasionally resort to other ventilation methods. Second, the effectiveness of gas exchange is higher than with other approaches, because the insufflation of gas occurs deeply in the airway. One drawback, however, is the risk of accidental

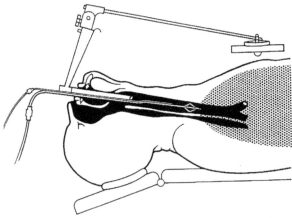

Fig. 1. Infraglottic jet ventilation setting with a double-lumen jet catheter, which is positioned outside of the suspension laryngoscope.

air trapping in case of inadvertent closure of the gas egress pathway (unless the catheter is placed inside the lumen of an ETT). For the same reason, this technique is contraindicated if there is an upper airway obstruction. Basically, no catheter should be introduced through an airway narrowing when the remaining cross section for exhalation is less than 50% of normal. In these cases, the passage of the narrowing is permitted only with a rigid endoscope (**Fig. 2**); the jet nozzle has to be kept proximal to the narrowing.

Supraglottic Jet Ventilation

The supraglottic JV configuration is present when the jet nozzle is located proximal of (above) the vocal cord level, and the air stream is directed to some extent from the distance toward the glottis. For this purpose, modified suspension laryngoscopes (**Fig. 3**) with multiple channels are used.[3] One advantage of the supraglottic JV is that the larynx remains completely free of tubing, thus offering maximal visibility and accessibility for the surgeon. Another advantage is the higher security against lung

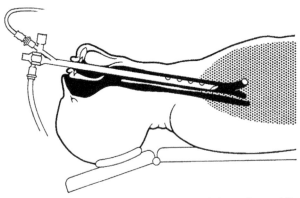

Fig. 2. Rigid bronchoscope connected at its proximal end through an oblique side port to the jet line of the ventilator.

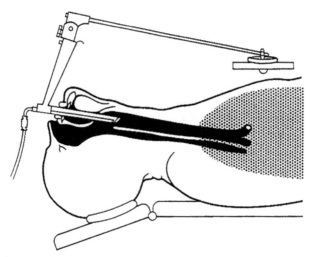

Fig. 3. Supraglottic JV through a dedicated lumen of a suspension laryngoscope.

injury, because the jet nozzle is located proximal of a possible obstruction. This could be the case of a closed glottis after diminishing of muscle relaxation. This feature makes this technology the first choice for JV in airway obstruction.[4] Alternatively, supraglottic JV is less efficient than the infraglottic variant, although this may be partially compensated by higher working pressure (WP) settings. It is important that the air stream is aligned axially to the open lumen of the airway. Another disadvantage of this procedure is that the ventilation can be installed only after the suspension laryngoscope has been correctly positioned. The same is true for emergence from anesthesia, when the spatula is removed at the end of the surgery. There have been also concerns that oncogenic or infectious particles (eg, papillomas) can be dragged distally into the airways. This conjecture has plausibility, but such a complication has not yet been observed or demonstrated.

Transtracheal Jet Ventilation

A transtracheal JV is present when the gas insufflation is performed through a transtracheal catheter. This is a short, very narrow (1.0 mm ID) and single-lumen catheter, which is passed through the skin and the cricothyroid ligament (or the space beneath the cricoid and above the first tracheal cartilage). The tip of the catheter is axially aligned and pointing downward into the subglottic region of the trachea (**Fig. 4**). This technique can be applied in cases of difficult or impossible laryngoscopy. For this reason, the transtracheal JV is suitable as a rescue oxygenation technique in the so-called cannot intubate–cannot ventilate scenario or in cases of imminent asphyxia.[5] Some centers even apply transtracheal JV in elective procedures as well.[6,7] The placement of the transtracheal catheter, however, is difficult and may bear severe complications; therefore, this technique should be used in a strictly standardized mode by users who have practiced first on phantoms or cadavers. Absolutely essential in this application is the need for an unobstructed opening for the outflow of the jet gas via larynx and oral cavity. If the causative airway obstruction is so great that a threat of lung overexpansion is present, transtracheal JV is inappropriate, unless an additional releasing incision into the trachea is made. Because the indication (the threat of asphyxia) and contraindications (severe airway obstruction) for this method are close to each other, and the distinction is based more or less on the severity of the stenosis, this technique is predominantly

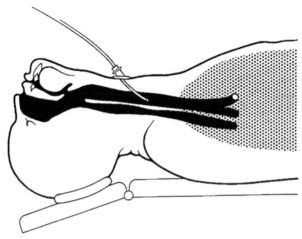

Fig. 4. Transtracheal JV via a Ravussin-type canula.

considered a last resort measure in emergency situations, and has to be performed by experienced users only.[8]

OPERATION MODES
Automatic Jet Ventilation Mode

An automatic JV mode is given if the device is electrically operated and if it applies the gas insufflations automatically according to settings specified by the user. This is standard practice in JV.[9] Typical settings for an average adult person are WP 1.6 bar, ventilation frequency (VF) 150 cycles per minute (cpm), and inspiration/exhalation ratio 1:1. In automatic mode, the parameters set by the device are kept constant, except preset airway pressure (Paw) limits are exceeded, which should lead to automatic switch-off of the device. This mode is more convenient for users because both hands are free and constant ventilation performance can be presumed.

Manual Jet Ventilation Mode

In manual JV, each insufflated gas portion is triggered by pressing a button or a lever on the ventilator. The duration of insufflation and, hence, the applied gas volume are defined by the manual actuation of the lever. This can happen with both, manual activation with an automatic ventilator (as an application variant), as well as with a simple jet injector, which is operated solely by hand. This application form is more suitable for emergency ventilation situations—for example, in the context of an imminent asphyxia and attempt of transtracheal oxygenation or for shorter periods of time in terms of a bridging measure until a definitive method of airway securing and oxygenation is applied. Typically, manually administered JV is performed as a low-frequency JV with approximately 20 cpm.[10] With low VF, the resulting longer insufflation duration leads to higher gas volumes, which are associated with a higher risk for lung overdistention. Therefore, manual insufflations should start generally with a very low WP (<0.8 bar) that can be gradually increased until visible chest excursions are noticed.

Superimposed Jet Ventilation

Superimposed high-frequency JV (SHFJV) is characterized by the simultaneous combination of two separate jet insufflation systems, one of which is operated with a high VF and another one with a low VF.[11] The two insufflation systems have a complementary and supra-additive effect on gas exchange efficiency. This may be of particular benefit in patients with significantly reduced lung function, when the traditional monofrequent JV becomes ineffective. Due to the necessity for two different nozzles, additional lines for Paw measurement and capnography, and even for smoke evacuation, this technique cannot be applied through an infraglottic or transtracheal catheter. SHFJV can be used either with a special suspension laryngoscope or through a special multilumen adapter for ETTs.

VENTILATION SETTINGS AND RESULTING PARAMETERS
Working Pressure

The WP is defined as the input pressure from the external gas source that is translated through the jet tubing reaching to the nozzle. A jet ventilator does not generate the WP actively; it only interrupts the continuous gas flow and allows an adjusted reduction of the output pressure. Thus, the WP is always lower than the inlet pressure of the external gas source. The WP is the setting with the greatest influence on the efficiency of gas exchange.[12] There is no linear correlation between the WP and any gas exchange parameters. Changes of WP produce nonproportional changes in the insufflated gas volume.[1]

Ventilation Frequency

The VF is the number of cycles generated per time. Usually the VF is initially set at approximately 150 cpm, but in certain conditions this might vary from 12 to 300 cpm. As a tendency, higher frequencies allow a smoother working field for surgeons, because the amplitude of tidal movements of the vocal cords and the operating field are smaller, but when increasing the VF, the proportion of dead space ventilation increases also, which might reduce the efficiency of CO_2 elimination.[13] Oxygenation is largely independent of the VF. The higher the VF is set, the more likely there is an auto–positive end-expiratory pressure (auto-PEEP), which builds up rapidly if the exhalation time duration is shortened. Due to the existing resistance of the exhalation pathway, the gas egress becomes hampered and the auto-PEEP might reach undesired values.[14] This in turn may have a relatively minor beneficial impact on oxygenation and an undesirable increase in the intrathoracic pressure. In infraglottic JV, the VF can be deliberately increased at the end of surgery and during emergence from anesthesia up to 300 cpm. Jet ventilators that are marketed in the United States are not approved for frequencies above 150 cpm. Setting the oxygen concentration to 100% and the WP to 0.8 bar achieves an almost continuous flow of oxygen, thus practically enabling a so-called apnoeic oxygenation but little CO_2 elimination. Patients may at any time breathe spontaneously, because the JV does not interfere with breathing. This makes the transition from JV to wakefulness easy without the necessity of intubation and conventional mechanical ventilation.

Inspiration Duration

The concept of ID has been adopted from conventional ventilation; more precisely, it defines the time ratio between active insufflation and passive exhalation. During the latter, insufflation is simply halted. Accordingly, the ID value is best presented as percentage of the insufflation time in relation to a whole respiratory cycle. The default value is usually set at 50%. In contrast changes of ID in conventional ventilation, modifications of the ID in JV have an immediate effect on the delivered gas volumes. Longer ID, therefore, leads to a shorter pause duration, which hinders exhalation and increases the auto-PEEP.[15] These effects in turn are heavily dependent on the VF; so, no blanket statements can be made for quantitative changes of ID. There is a trend for slight improvement of oxygenation by extending the ID, but this happens at the expense of CO_2 elimination. Secondarily, there is a shift of the thoracic excursions into a deeper inspiratory position, which in turn can lead to higher Paws and consequently worsen gas exchange as well. In general, modifications of the ID are usually followed by changes in other parameters and the resulting effects on gas exchange are rather unpredictable. Therefore, it does not make sense to vary the ID; it seems to be the best to keep it at or near by 50%.[9]

Oxygen Concentration in the Jet Gas

The oxygen fraction in the jet gas ($Fjeto_2$) results from the mixture of O_2 and air, which is supplied from the high-pressure gas sources to the gas mixer. The fraction of oxygen can be varied between 0.21 (air) and 1.0 (pure oxygen). It is natural to equate the $Fjeto_2$ with the inspiratory oxygen concentration as used in conventional ventilation. But this analogy is not correct, because due to air entrainment, the incoming oxygen concentration in the airway inevitably decreases below the set $Fjeto_2$ value. The higher the $Fjeto_2$ is set, the more pronounced is this effect. Also, the magnitude of entrainment is highly dependent on the configuration of the ventilation equipment. The more distal the jet nozzle is located in the respiratory tract, the less ambient air is in its vicinity, and the local oxygen concentration is less affected. The negative impact of entrainment is that of lowering the available oxygen concentration. This undesired effect can be attenuated by a separate insufflation of oxygen into the vicinity of the jet nozzle (so-called bias flow). Although an increase in the $Fjeto_2$ is the most likely measure to improve oxygenation, its reduction is a desirable objective in the application of laser beams. Even by meticulously avoiding ignitable material, and exclusively using laser-resistant equipment, a residual risk of ignition and fire complications remains.[16] This is due to particles released from the tissue of the operated patient, which can be ignited in an oxygen-rich atmosphere. To keep this risk to a minimum, the lowest possible oxygen concentration in the ventilation gas (<40%) has to be observed during activation of the laser probe.[17]

Gas Volumes

A resulting parameter in JV is the volume of the delivered gas, expressed either as TV (TV = volume of one insufflation cycle) or minute volume (MV = TV · VF). In contrast to conventional ventilators, gas volumes in JV are not identical to the corresponding thoracic excursions. The volume of chest expansion is much smaller than the applied gas volumes, thus indicating that a large part of the delivered gas amount caused only a washout of the airways. Only a small part of the gas is translated to alveolar ventilation.[18,19] Furthermore, TV and MV are not set parameters but resulting ones, which are variable depending on multiple factors. The gas volumes are directly influenced by WP and ID as well as by the geometry of gas-carrying components and the airway itself. An increase in WP results in higher TV and MV; however, this relationship is not linear because of the complex interaction of multiple factors, such as resistance of the whole system and the morphology of the respiratory tract.

Airway Pressure

The Paw is also a resulting parameter and is influenced by various factors, mainly the WP. As long as no obstacle to the gas outflow exists, the Paw remains very low in the magnitude of a few millibars. VF and ID have little direct impact on the Paw, except in extreme settings when it comes to remarkable changes in gas volume. Additional factors, such as size and shape of the jet nozzle and the airway geometry, are involved.[20] Because high Paw directly bears the risk of lung distension and lung injury, a continuous measurement of Paw is required as is an automatic shutdown of ventilation if user-determined pressure limits are exceeded.[21] A state-of-the-art jet ventilator is equipped with a redundant Paw monitoring. Via a dedicated line, the Paw is continuously measured and displayed as a pressure curve indicating its main determinants, such as peak inspiratory pressure, mean Paw, and end-expiratory pressure. Separately, the pressure course is also measured in the jet tube, but because of technical reasons, this is only possible during the short break between the insufflations. Here, another alarm limit is set (break pressure), which needs to be undercut during each cycle so that the next insufflation can be released. For this kind of double-Paw monitoring, correspondingly, a jet catheter with 2 lumens is required. The measured Paw in the trachea is not identical to the Paws in various portions of the lung but may be accepted as a good approximation. This can be used to activate the necessary alarms and to respect the pressure limits determined by the user.

Monitoring

Because JV is characterized by an open breathing system, the compositions of the insufflated and exhaled gas cannot be directly assessed.[21] These parameters remain in the routine clinical application ultimately unknown. Only the quantities and composition of gas delivered by the device are shown. The standard equipment includes the delivered oxygen concentration and the resulting Paw course.

The patient parameters of gas exchange are pulse oximetry, capnography, and sometimes invasive arterial or noninvasive transcutaneous blood gas measurements. Although monitoring oxygenation poses no major difficulties, the surveillance of the CO_2 status is technically more demanding because of the lack of direct and exclusive access to the exhaled gas. The monitoring of CO_2 elimination is an important task in JV to adjust the ventilator settings according to the actual gas exchange status. Intermittent arterial blood gas sampling provides only selective information and, moreover, is dependent on the presence of an arterial line. Therefore, this method is inappropriate for the vast majority of cases and should be considered for long interventions in morbid patients only.

Capnometry requires a separate access to the airway, which is possible, for example, with multilumen jet catheters, tube adapters, or suspension laryngoscopes, where a dedicated channel for gas sampling is available.[22] When a gas sample is aspirated through an intratracheally lying catheter, there is a risk that this line is going to be obstructed with mucus or blood. Additionally, the capnography signal, which is acquired during high-frequency JV, is not quantitative, because the response of the CO_2 electrode is too slow to reach the end-tidal value before the next cycle washes the sample away. Therefore, the capnogram shows only a saw tooth-like curve with a small amplitude, which can serve only as an indication of the integrity of the ventilation.[23] To determine the CO_2 status, switch intermittently to low-frequency JV, so that an end-tidal CO_2 ($EtCO_2$) value can be measured and displayed. An alternative is the measurement of transcutaneous PCO_2 ($Ptcco_2$), which also provides useful results in adults.[24] Its sensor requires a warm-up period of several minutes, which does not matter if it is placed at the beginning of anesthesia as a first measure. Another limitation is the latency period of approximately 1 minute. Because the CO_2 production is not more than 0.5 kPa per minute, this delay does not cause a problem in terms of adjusting the JV according the CO_2 status.[25] The limited accuracy of transcutaneous CO_2 measurement is also a point of criticism. Generally speaking, we have to admit that in contrast to capnometry, transcutaneous measurement is local only. It does not represent a global value of the whole organism, but it yields a fair trend of the global CO_2 course and is, therefore, suitable for adjusting the ventilation. The difference between transcutaneous measuerement results on the one hand, and capnometric and arterial sample results on the other ranges usually between 0.5 and 1.5 kPa. The main advantage of $Ptcco_2$ is that it is noninvasive, continuous, simple to handle, and independent of the breathing system. For adjustment of the ventilation, it is sufficient to observe the trend of $Ptcco_2$ and to compare it with the baseline value under spontaneous breathing before induction of anesthesia.[26]

Jet Gas Conditioning

Prolonged ventilation with unconditioned (dry and cold) ventilation gas may cause damage to the tracheobronchial mucosa.[27] This can range from a temporary disturbance of mucociliary clearance with risk of subsequent infection to a life-threatening necrotizing tracheobronchitis.[28] In addition to the duration of ventilation, other predisposing factors are known, such as circulatory instability, physical pressure on the mucosa, and pre-existing mucosal damage, as is the case in smokers. The combination of these factors makes it impossible to identify a safe duration of application without gas conditioning, which makes popular estimations, such as less than 30 minutes, at least questionable. Less dangerous, but also undesirable, is the immediately occurring hypothermia during unconditioned JV. This is not surprising considering large quantities of gas (20–30 L/min) that are injected directly in the immediate vicinity of the large thoracic vessels, thus representing an efficient heat exchanger. After 15 minutes of unconditioned JV, a drop in body core temperature of up to 2°C is possible.[21]

Ideal conditioning means that the jet gas is heated to 37°C and enriched with 100% relative humidity before it leaves the nozzle. A heating of the jet gas without humidification is inefficient due to the fact that dry gas has a much-reduced capacity to transport heat. This way it also dries the mucosa even more. Conversely, a sole water supply without heating is hardly a viable humidification; it would be simply a useless and possibly harmful intratracheal water infusion.

There are physical limits in gas conditioning that have to be taken into account. At the level of the jet nozzle, there is a huge drop in pressure, which causes an expansion of the jet gas. The latter is associated with a loss in energy and consequently in a loss of heat and humidity-bearing capacity. The maximum moisture loading of gas is 44 mg/L at 37°C, whereas at 22°C this is only 19 mg/L. The result of this is that moistened jet gas contains amounts of condensed water in the form of water droplets of various sizes. These in turn do not contribute to conditioning. The water droplets are injected into the respiratory tract, where they are rapidly absorbed. The resulting volume of absorbed water depends on the MV, the set humidification level, and can amount to several hundred milliliters per hour. A part is removed with the exhaled gas, but the rest can be counted as unintended infusion. Because for humidification only distilled water may be used, there is a slow but continuous systemic supply of free water, which, in case of long-lasting application, affects the fluid balance and plasma osmolarity status. Theoretically, it is possible to reduce the amount of condensation using a heated jet line, but this is technically complex and yields undesirable risks due to the proximity of electrical equipment to the patient. The currently usual equipment is designed so that the heat is added to the gas in the jet ventilator at 100°C and moistened to the set level. Then it is accepted that the gas cools to 37°C over the predetermined length of the jet line, and the remaining condensation of a portion of the gas humidity is accepted as unavoidable.

The conditioning level may be gradually regulated from 0 to 100%, which is not to be confused with relative or absolute humidity percentage. This conditioning level is a combination of moisture supply and heating, whereas the output power is automatically adjusted to the supplied gas volume (MV). The higher the power is set, the greater is the proportion of the condensate. In settings under 100%, a part of the moisture can be maintained despite the cooling of the gas. The essential message for the user is that one should always work with the maximum possible conditioning to ensure the best tolerance of JV. A disadvantage of high-performance conditioning is, however, that a surgeon's laser microscope can be blurred by the exhaled water vapor. Only this case is a justified reason to reduce the gas conditioning step by step to the extent that the visual disability is avoided for a restricted duration of time.

COMMON PROBLEMS WITH JET VENTILATION
Insufficient Oxygenation

Problems with oxygenation are occasionally observed, and then they appear in two forms. A sudden drop in saturation may be the result of an acute pneumothorax. This should be quickly verified and treated by thoracic drainage. A slow decline in saturation is usually due to insufficient ventilation or limited pulmonary diffusion capacity. Behind these cases, there is usually a combined restrictive-obstructive pneumopathy, mostly associated with a significant reduction in vital capacity. A whole series of technical measures can counteract the gradual decline in oxygen saturation. First, the oxygen concentration in the jet gas should be increased. If this measure is exhausted without achieving the desired success, the WP can be increased. Further steps to improve oxygenation may include the extending the ID, reducing the ambient air entrainment (by adding an O_2 bias flow), or switching from supraglottic to the more efficient infraglottic JV.[21] If these measures are exhausted and still no adequate oxygenation is achieved, there remains the alternative of intermittent conventional ventilation or switching entirely to positive pressure ventilation.

Insufficient CO_2 Elimination

Hypercapnia can be observed in patients with predominantly obstructive pneumopathy (chronic obstructive pulmonary disease).[25] Often these are obese individuals with reduced thoracic compliance. The technical possibility for counteracting a continual rise in the $Paco_2$ is to increase the WP up to the available technical limits. The necessary WP level can be determined by assessing the resulting $Paco_2$ after stepwise increasing of the WP until the $Paco_2$ surge stops. An upper limitation of the WP is given only from the available pressure of the gas sources, which are usually in the range of 4.0 to 4.5 bar. In patients who are ventilated with the maximally available WP, and in whom $Paco_2$ rises further, it has to be decided which degree of hypercapnia is tolerable. From available experience, it can be assumed that an increase of $Paco_2$ to the extent of 1.5 times baseline can be tolerated at the end of surgery. At that point, the CO_2 status can be normalized by intermittent or definitive switch to conventional ventilation via an ETT or a laryngeal mask.[29]

EQUIPMENT

Anesthesia working places where JV is used have to be fully equipped with a conventional anesthesia system—preferably containing a regular anesthesia ventilator—that is, mainly used for induction and emergence from anesthesia, but which also is an essential backup device for the case that JV proves to be insufficient. Basic monitoring of heart rate, noninvasive blood pressure, pulse oximetry, and capnometry is also mandatory. Because the market for jet ventilators is not large, only a few different devices are marketed. The two recently available high-end jet ventilators are the Monsoon III Universal Jet Ventilator (Acutronic MS, Hirzel, Switzerland) and the Twin

Stream (Carl Rainer, Vienna, Austria). Both systems are equipped with various setting options and have comfortable reading of parameters on their display. The more recent Monsoon III, however, has an integrated gas conditioning system, which permits its use for unlimited time durations. Additionally, the Monsoon III has an integrated capnography unit, which can be programmed to automatically perform five consecutive low-frequency insufflations to achieve a readable end-tidal CO_2 signal. In many places, several precursors of these machines are still in use and might be operated under the condition that safety conditions are met. These are the older Monsoon versions (I and II), the Mistral UJV, and the AMS 1000 (Acutronic MS, Hirzel, Switzerland).

A simple and low-cost manual jet ventilator is the ManuJet (VBM, Sulz am Neckar, Germany) that is designed to be used for emergency (transtracheal) jet oxygenation and ventilation. This device can also be used for very short elective procedures, but it is not recommended as standard equipment in upper airway surgery. For the transtracheal access to the airway, a Ravussin-type cricothyrotomy catheter can be used, which has one lumen and an outer diameter of 1.3 mm (VBM, Sulz am Neckar, Germany).

To monitor oxygenation, pulse oximetry can be relied on. The surveillance of the CO_2 status is more demanding and necessitates either the intermittent low-frequency feature of the Monsoon III or the use of a separate capnography unit for which the ventilation has to be altered manually. Transcutaneous CO_2 measurement is a feasible alternative, but it necessitates the availability of an additional device, such as the MicroGas 7650 with a combined P_{O_2} and P_{CO_2} electrode or the TCM TOSCA (Radiometer Medical ApS, Brønshøj, Denmark) with a combined S_{PO_2} and P_{CO_2} sensor. Another versatile transcutaneous blood gas monitor is the SenTec Digital Monitor (Sentec AG, Therwil, Switzerland). For features, benefits, and limitations of transcutaneous blood gas monitoring, see previous discussion of "Monitoring."

ACKNOWLEDGMENTS

The author has been involved in development of jet ventilation–related equipment manufactured by Acutronic MS (Hirzel, Switzerland) and VBM (Sulz am Neckar, Germany) and mentioned in this article.

REFERENCES

1. Aloy A, Schragl E. Jet-ventilation. Technische grundlagen und klinische anwendungen. NewYork: Springer; 1995.
2. Frochaux D, Rajan GP, Biro P. [Laser-resistance of a new jet ventilation catheter (LaserJet) under simulated clinical conditions]. Anaesthesist 2004;53:820–5 [in German].
3. Schragl E, Donner A, Kashanipour A, et al. [Preliminary experiences with superimpoposed high-frequence jet ventilation in intensive care]. Anaesthesist 1995; 44:429 [in German].
4. Schragl E, Donner A, Kashanipour A, et al. [Anesthesia in acute respiratory tract obstructions caused by high degree laryngeal and tracheobronchial stenoses]. Anasthesiol Intensivmed Notfallmed Schmerzther 1994;29:269–77 [in German].
5. Hamaekers AE, Gotz T, Borg PA, et al. Achieving an adequate minute volume through a 2 mm transtracheal catheter in simulated upper airway obstruction using a modified industrial ejector. Br J Anaesth 2010;104:382–6.
6. Biro P, Moe KS. Emergency transtracheal jet ventilation in high grade airway obstruction. J Clin Anesth 1997;9:604–7.

7. Scrase I, Woollard M. Needle vs surgical cricothyroidotomy: a short cut to effective ventilation. Anaesthesia 2006;61:962–74.

8. Kleemann PP. [Die schwierige intubation]. Anaesthesist 1996;45:1248–67 [in German].

9. Biro P, Wiedemann K. [Jet ventilation and anaesthesia for diagnostic and therapeutic interventions of the airway]. Anaesthesist 1999;48:669–85 [in German].

10. Bould MD, Bearfield P. Techniques for emergency ventilation through a needle cricothyroidotomy. Anaesthesia 2008;63:535–9.

11. Ihra G, Kepka A, Lanzenberger E, et al. [SHFJV. Jet-adapter zur durchführung der superponierten hochfrequenz jet-ventilation über einen tubus in der intensivmedizin: eine technische neuerung]. Anaesthesist 1998;47:209–19 [in German].

12. Takahashi H, Takezawa J, Nishijima MK, et al. Effects of driving pressure and respiratory rate on airway pressure and $PaCO_2$ in rabbits during high-frequency jet ventilation. Crit Care Med 1985;13:728–32.

13. Young JD. Gas movement during jet ventilation. Acta Anaesthesiol Scand 1989; 33(Suppl 90):72–4.

14. Myles PS, Evans AB, Madder H, et al. Dynamic hyperinflation: comparison of jet ventilation versus conventional ventilation in patients with severe end-stage obstructive lung disease. Anaesth Intensive Care 1997;25:471–5.

15. Guenard H, Cros AM, Boundey C. Variations in flow and intraalveolar pressure during jet ventilation: theoretical and experimental analysis. Respir Physiol 1989;75:235–45.

16. Dhar V, Young K, Nouraei SA, et al. Impact of oxygen concentration and laser power on occurrence of intraluminal fires during shared-airway surgery: an investigation. J Laryngol Otol 2008;122:1335–8.

17. Juri O, Frochaux D, Rajan GP, et al. [Ignition and burning of biological tissue under simulated CO2-laser surgery conditions]. Anaesthesist 2006;55:541–6 [in German].

18. Gaughan SD, Ozaki GT, Benumof JL. A comparison in a lung model of low- and high-flow regulators for transtracheal jet ventilation. Anesthesiology 1992;77: 189–99.

19. Lichtwarck-Aschoff M, Zimmermann GJ, Erhardt W. Reduced CO2-elimination during combined high-frequency ventilation compared to conventional pressure-controlled ventilation in surfactant-deficient piglets. Acta Anaesthesiol Scand 1998;42:335–42.

20. van Vught AJ, Versprille A, Jansen JR. Alveolar pressure during high-frequency jet ventilation. Intensive Care Med 1990;16:33–40.

21. Biro P, Schmid S. [Anesthesia and high frequency jet ventilation (HFJV) for surgical interventions on the larynx and trachea]. HNO 1997;45:43–52 [in German].

22. Baer GA, Paloheimo M, Rahnasto J, et al. End-tidal oxygen concentration and pulse oximetry for monitoring oxygenation during intratracheal jet ventilation. J Clin Monit 1995;11:373–80.

23. Klein U, Gottschall R, Hannemann U, et al. [Capnography for bronchoscopy with rigid technique using high frequency jet ventilation (HFJV)]. Anasthesiol Intensivmed Notfallmed Schmerzther 1995;30:276–82 [in German].

24. Biro P, Rohling R, Weiss BM. High-frequency jet-ventilation in adult surgical patients monitored by transcutaneous PCO2-measurements. Br J Anaesth 1996;76(Suppl 2):20.

25. Biro P, Eyrich G, Rohling R. The efficiency of CO2 elimination during high-frequency jet ventilation for laryngeal microsurgery. Anesth Analg 1998;87:180–4.

26. Atkins JH, Mirza N, Mandel JE. Case report: respiratory inductance plethysmography as a monitor of ventilation during laser ablation and balloon dilatation of subglottic tracheal stenosis. ORL J Otorhinolaryngol Relat Spec 2009;71:289–91.

27. Dias NH, Martins RH, Braz JR, et al. Larynx and cervical trachea in humidification and heating of inhaled gases. Ann Otol Rhinol Laryngol 2005;114:411–5.

28. Doyle HJ, Napolitano AE, Lippmann HR, et al. Different humidification systems for high-frequency jet-ventilation. Crit Care Med 1984;12:815–9.

29. Gentz BA, Shupak RC, Bhatt SB, et al. Carbon dioxide dynamics during apneic oxygenation: the effects of preceding hypocapnia. J Clin Anesth 1998;10:189–94.

Anesthetic Considerations for Transoral Robotic Surgery

John J. Chi, MD[a],*, Jeff E. Mandel, MD, MS[b],
Gregory S. Weinstein, MD[a], Bert W. O'Malley Jr, MD[a]

KEYWORDS

- TORS • Transoral robotic surgery • Head and neck cancer
- Tonsil cancer • Larynx cancer • Da Vinci surgical system

During the past decade, robotic surgery has been progressively incorporated into the mainstream of cardio-thoracic and abdomino-pelvic surgery. With the recent US Food and Drug Administration (FDA) approval of transoral robotic surgery (TORS) for the treatment of all benign tumors and select malignant tumors of the head and neck, robotic surgery has established its place in otolaryngologic surgery. Given the multi-specialty applications and widespread use of robotic surgery, there exists a need for anesthesiologists to familiarize themselves with robotic surgery. This article focuses on TORS and the goal of which is to provide the anesthesiologist with a foundation for caring for the TORS patient in the perioperative period.

TRANSORAL ROBOTIC SURGERY

TORS is a minimally invasive surgical technique, first developed by Weinstein and O'Malley.[1–7] Through their early investigations of feasibility using the daVinci Surgical Robot (Intuitive Surgical, Sunnyvale, CA, USA), they found that TORS was most effective if performed through mouth gags rather than traditional laryngoscopes. Further studies of patient safety ultimately led to the first application of TORS in human patients. Currently, TORS is performed by otolaryngologists throughout the United States and the number continues to grow as more and more surgeons become trained in TORS techniques.

TORS with the daVinci Surgical Robot addresses several key challenges inherent to otolaryngologic surgery. Like sternotomies in cardiac surgery and laparotomies in

[a] Department of Otorhinolaryngology–Head & Neck Surgery, University of Pennsylvania School of Medicine, 3400 Spruce Street, 5 Ravdin, Philadelphia, PA 19104, USA
[b] Department of Anesthesiology & Critical Care, University of Pennsylvania School of Medicine, 3400 Spruce Street, Philadelphia, PA 19104, USA
* Corresponding author.
E-mail address: john.chi@uphs.upenn.edu

Anesthesiology Clin 28 (2010) 411–422
doi:10.1016/j.anclin.2010.07.002   **anesthesiology.theclinics.com**
1932-2275/10/$ – see front matter © 2010 Elsevier Inc. All rights reserved.

urologic surgery, otolaryngologic surgery often mandates surgical exposures that are far greater than the surgical field that the tissues are manipulated within. TORS allows the otolaryngologist true 3-dimensional endoscopic vision of the surgical field with accurate depth perception through the use of multiple endoscopes, cameras, and dual eye pieces. TORS supplants the limited visualization of the 2-dimensional endoscope and line-of-sight microscope. The limitations of traditional laparoscopic and endoscopic instrument manipulation are also improved on in TORS. The robotic system allows multiple degrees of motion (flexion, extension, supination, pronation) and through robotic scaling transforms large movements of the surgeon's hands into small movements of the robotic instruments. The tremor of the human hand is also filtered through the use of a robotic system resulting in smooth bimanual dexterity within the surgical field.[8] When compared with standard open surgical approaches, TORS offers significant potential benefits to patients. TORS use may avoid a disfiguring mandibulotomy, tracheostomy, and minimize or possibly eliminate the need for chemoradiation therapy. Additionally, decreased blood loss, risk of wound infection, and postoperative pain allows for a shorter recovery time with a quicker return to preoperative speech, swallowing, and quality of life.[6,7]

PREOPERATIVE ASSESSMENT

The FDA has approved the daVinci surgical system for all benign lesions of the oral cavity, larynx, and pharynx and all T1 and T2 malignancies and has excluded all pediatric disease and lesions that invade the mandible. Dental procedures are also excluded. At the authors' institution, before performing TORS, the patient routinely undergoes panendoscopy (direct laryngoscopy, bronchoscopy, esophagoscopy). During the panendoscopy, TORS feasibility is assessed with regard to surgical exposure. Additionally, the lesion is biopsied for pathologic diagnosis to ensure that the patient meets appropriate surgical indications for TORS. An added benefit of this process is the opportunity for the anesthesiologist to meet the patient in the context of a minimally invasive, brief procedure before undertaking subsequent more invasive procedures. This improves the efficiency of use of time booked with the daVinci robot.

OPERATING ROOM SETUP

The operating surgeon is located at the surgeon's console approximately 10 feet away from the patient (**Fig. 1**). The surgical assistant is located at the patient's head and assists with suction and retraction. The anesthesiologist and anesthesia machine are located at the patient's feet. The nurse and instrument carts are located on the side of the patient opposite the surgeon to minimize obstruction and maximize communication between surgeon, assistant, and anesthesiologist. The daVinci Surgical Robot consists of a master surgeon's console, a surgical cart, and a robotic patient-side cart. The robotic patient-side cart has 3 robotic arms—2 laterally placed arms, which hold instruments, and a centrally placed arm for the endoscopic camera (**Fig. 2**). The 2 instrument arms hold interchangeable instruments with miniaturized versions of standard surgical instruments, such as electrocautery and forceps (**Fig. 3**).

At the beginning of a TORS case, the patient is placed in the supine position and the airway is secured using standard endotracheal intubation. This may be accomplished before or subsequent to rotation of the patient 180 degrees away from the anesthesiologist. Although induction in the rotated position requires planning and assistance, it may significantly reduce induction time, as the patient-side cart can be set up before induction. The patient is then draped in the standard fashion for transoral otolaryngologic surgery. During all TORS cases the patient's eyes are protected using plastic

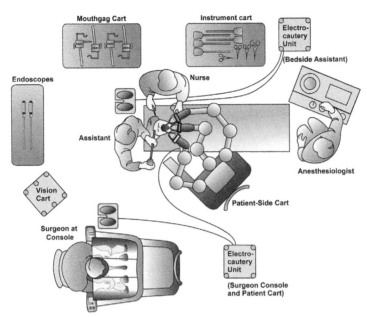

Fig. 1. Operating room setup. (*Courtesy of* Intuitive Surgical, Inc., Sunnyvale, CA. © 2008 Intuitive Surgical, Inc.)

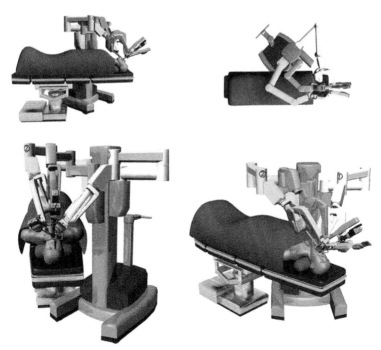

Fig. 2. Patient with robotic patient-side cart. (*Courtesy of* Intuitive Surgical, Inc., Sunnyvale, CA. © 2008 Intuitive Surgical, Inc.)

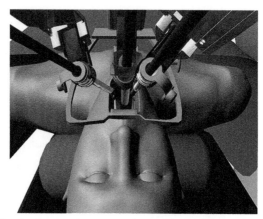

Fig. 3. Patient with robotic arms. (*Courtesy of* Intuitive Surgical, Inc., Sunnyvale, CA. © 2008 Intuitive Surgical, Inc.)

patient safety goggles and the teeth are protected with a molded dental guard. The endotracheal tube is routinely sutured to the patient's face by the operating surgeon for airway stability. Endotracheal tube selection is dependent on the TORS being performed. If tumor resection encroaches upon the larynx or pyriform sinus, then a laser endotracheal tube is used, otherwise a wire-reinforced endotracheal tube is used. If the case involves the use of an operating laser, then standard patient safety measures should be implemented (covering the head and neck with moistened towels, taping and covering the patient's eyes, eye protection for operating room personnel, laser endotracheal tube, and so forth). Next, if not already in position, the robotic patient-side cart is brought into position at a 30° angle to the operating room table. This configuration allows for introduction of the 3 robotic arms through the mouth and into the patient's upper airway.

The operating surgeon then places a mouth gag or retractor in the patient to gain surgical exposure. Then, the 3 sterilely draped robotic arms are placed into surgical position. At this point, the operating room personnel assume the configuration seen in **Fig. 1** and the surgery commences. After the completion of the surgical resection, hemostasis is achieved using bipolar cautery and hemoclips with confirmation of a bloodless surgical field via the Valsalva maneuver. Next, a final assessment of the airway is made by the surgical team. If there is significant laryngopharyngeal edema or concern that airway compromise might develop, then the wire-reinforced or Laser-Flex tube (Mallinckrodt, Hazelwood, MO, USA) is exchanged for a polyvinyl chloride (PVC) tube and the patient is extubated only after resolution of the edema. Following airway evaluation, the robotic arms, dental guard, and mouth gag or retractor are removed from the patient. The robotic patient-side cart is pulled away from the operating room table and the patient is returned to the anesthesiologist for extubation.

Tissue removal is accomplished with monopolar cautery and bipolary cautery, as well as flexible carbon dioxide laser.[9–11]

TORS PROCEDURES

Similar to other new surgical procedures, operating room times for TORS can initially be substantial. Genden and colleagues[11] reported up to 140 minutes of robotic setup time for one of the early TORS cases performed at their institution. Fortunately, the learning curve is steep. The preoperative setup time dramatically decreases as surgical experience increases.[6,7,11–13] Moore and colleagues[13] reported that after only 10 TORS cases, the preoperative setup time dropped from approximately 69 minutes to 22 minutes. Although operative experience also improves operative time, Moore and colleagues[13] found that operative time was highly dependent on the tumor burden present at the time of resection—not unlike other oncologic surgery. Mean overall operative times are reported in **Table 1**.

Radical Tonsillectomy

The TORS radical tonsillectomy is a modification of the transoral lateral oropharyngectomy described by Holsinger and colleagues.[14] An oral endotracheal tube is sutured to both the contralateral nasolabial fold and the buccal mucosa. A Crow-Davis mouth gag is used to gain surgical exposure. The 0° video endoscope is used for this procedure. Using monopolar electrocautery, an incision is made through the buccal mucosa and a plane is developed along the lateral aspect of the pharyngeal constrictor muscles. The plane is carried medial to the pterygoid musculature to the level of the styloglossus and stylopharyngeus muscles. Next, the soft palate is transected to the level of the prevertebral fascia followed by elevation of the constrictor muscles off of the prevertebral fascia to the level of the styloglossus and stylopharyngeus muscles. The styloglossus and stylopharyngeus muscles are then bluntly dissected circumferentially and then carefully transected. The carotid arterial system runs in the region of this dissection and special care must be taken to avoid dissecting near these vessels. Branches of the tonsillar and ascending pharyngeal vessels are routinely encountered and ligated with cautery or hemoclips. The dissection proceeds to the tongue base with an incision across the posterior floor of mouth mucosa to the lateral tongue base mucosa. Then, the tongue base musculature is transected for a clear margin around the tumor. Additional effort must be made to avoid inadvertently transecting the lingual artery during this dissection, as bleeding can be brisk. The

Table 1 Operative times for TORS			
Institution	TORS Procedure	No. of Patients	Mean Overall Operative Time, Min
University of Pennsylvania[6]	Base of tongue resection	3	148
University of Pennsylvania[12]	Supraglottic partial laryngectomy	3	122
University of Pennsylvania[7]	Radical tonsillectomy	27	103
Mayo Clinic[13]	Radical tonsillectomy, base of tongue resection	45	104
Mount Sinai[11]	Radical tonsillectomy, base of tongue resection, supraglottic partial laryngectomy, partial pharyngectomy	18	139
University of Pavia, University of Pisana[22]	Base of tongue resection for obstructive sleep apnea	10	87

Abbreviation: TORS, transoral robotic surgery.

tongue base is resected to the level of the vallecula. The posterior pharyngeal wall is then resected from the vallecula to the soft palate, completing the surgical resection.

Base of Tongue Resection

The TORS base of tongue resection uses the principle of en bloc tumor resection for maximal oncologic control contrary to other transoral surgical approaches that use piecemeal resection of the base of tongue. An oral endotracheal tube is sutured to both the contralateral nasolabial fold and the buccal mucosa. A Crow-Davis mouth gag or Feyh-Kastenbauer (FK) laryngeal retractor is used to gain surgical exposure. Both the 0° and 30° video endoscopes are used for this procedure. Using monopolar electrocautery, an incision is made in the anterior and medial base of tongue mucosa. As in the radical tonsillectomy, tongue musculature is resected for a clear margin around the tumor and care is taken to avoid the lingual artery. The dissection continues in the lateral base of tongue and is carried to the vallecula. The vallecular mucosa is then freed from the epiglottis and the tongue base is transected from the lateral pharyngeal wall, completing the surgical resection.

Supraglottic Partial Laryngectomy

The TORS partial laryngectomy is a modification of the transoral supraglottic partial laryngectomy described by Rudert and colleagues.[15] A wire-reinforced oral endotracheal tube is sutured to both the contralateral nasolabial fold and the buccal mucosa. An FK laryngeal retractor is used to gain surgical exposure. Both the 0° and 30° video endoscopes are used for this procedure. Using a monopolar cautery, the epiglottis is divided in the midline to the level of the petiole. Given the proximity of electrocautery to the endotracheal tube, a wire-reinforced endotracheal tube must be used for this procedure. The dissection continues along the vallecular mucosa down one side of the supraglottis. After careful palpation and identification of the thyroid cartilage and hyoid bone, the supraglottis is dissected from the internal aspect of these structures. The superior laryngeal vessels are routinely encountered at this point in the dissection and ligated with cautery or hemoclips. The dissection continues through the aryepiglottic fold and false vocal cord with division of the lateral ventricular mucosa completing the surgical resection.

ANESTHETIC MANAGEMENT

Anesthetic management of TORS has similarities to transoral cases such as tonsillectomy and laser excision of laryngeal lesions, but there are significant points of departure. First, the patient is turned 180° away from the anesthesia machine. Second, a fairly large device, the daVinci surgical cart, is placed in the vicinity of the patient's head. Third, the patient is placed in suspension laryngoscopy. Fourth, the surgeon sits out of view of the anesthesia team at the console. Fifth, the room lights are typically off. All of these factors make situational awareness more challenging. The intraoperative setup is illustrated in **Fig. 4**. Although anesthesiologists may be involved in planning the location of the anesthesia equipment in a robotic surgical suite, this almost certainly will be a room designed primarily for abdominal procedures, and access to the head when turned 180° may simply not have been considered.

As previously discussed, patients with advanced, extensive lesions with invasion of deep structures are not candidates for TORS. Preoperative x-ray therapy is rarely used. Thus, the likelihood of having difficult exposure at laryngoscopy is less than in the cohort of patients presenting for neck dissection for similar tumors. Additionally, in our practice, the vast majority of patients have undergone panendoscopy for

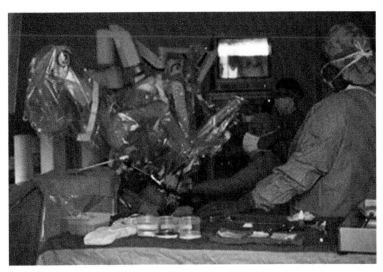

Fig. 4. Intraoperative position.

surgical planning. In our practice for panendoscopy, we use a technique in which the initial laryngoscopy is performed by the surgeon using a Lindholm or anterior commissure laryngoscope (Karl Storz, Germany) with high-frequency jet ventilation. When a question arises on the ability to intubate a patient at the time of TORS, the surgeon is available with a suspension laryngoscope, and intubation is performed with an endotracheal tube styletted with a 0° endoscope.[16] Other useful adjuncts include trans-laryngeal mask airway (LMA) intubation with the Aintree intubation catheter (Cook Medical, Bloomington, IN, USA)[17] and the GlideScope (Verathon, Bothell, WA, USA),[18] as illustrated in **Fig. 5**. Awake fiberoptic intubation is rarely used in our practice.

Endotracheal tube selection is typically a wire-reinforced tube, except in instances where the epiglottis will be divided, in which case a Laser-Flex tube is used.

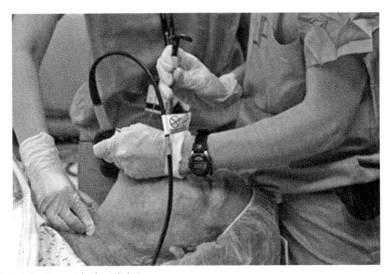

Fig. 5. Intubation with the GlideScope.

Anesthetic induction may be handled in conventional fashion; however, we commonly induce anesthesia with the bed turned 180° at the outset. This slightly complicates induction, but vastly simplifies the setup for the procedure. Following the induction, the robotic side cart must be brought in from the patient's right, and the endoscopy tower and scrub table must be brought in from the left. If the bed is to be rotated 180°, the preparation of these components must be deferred until after induction, rather than in parallel with induction. Turning the bed requires disconnecting and reconnecting monitors, intravenous (IV) lines, and the anesthesia circuit and rerouting these lines to avoid entanglement with the robot. By avoiding the bed turn, 15 to 20 minutes can be saved per case, permitting increased use of this expensive resource. It should be noted that the patient must be positioned with his or her head at the foot of the bed so that the pedestal of the bed is in the proper position when bringing the robotic cart into place. Performing an induction with the bed turned 180° requires some adjustment in technique. We typically use total intravenous anesthesia (TIVA), and use infusion pumps for propofol, remifentanil, and phenylepherine. The pump is positioned so that the anesthesiologist can easily access it during induction, and then turn it back to the position needed for maintenance, as illustrated in **Fig. 6**. The pumps are programmed to deliver an induction bolus followed by a maintenance infusion, providing a stable plane of anesthesia in the induction period. The anesthesia machine is used to deliver 100% oxygen with pressure-cycled ventilation at a pressure limit of 18 cm H_2O throughout the induction, and the anesthesia circuit is routed down the midline. This leaves the anesthetist with both hands free to perform jaw thrust during ventilation, as illustrated in **Fig. 7**. Two-handed mask ventilation using the ventilator has been described as a technique useful in patients predicted to be difficult to ventilate.[19] The anesthetist faces the anesthesia machine and monitors, permitting greater situational awareness during the induction. Additionally, there is no need to disconnect monitors during the postinduction period for the turn, eliminating a gap in vigilance during a period often characterized by hemodynamic instability.

We typically do not paralyze patients before intubation, as it reduces the ability to detect inadequate doses of TIVA and reduces our ability to back out of a difficult

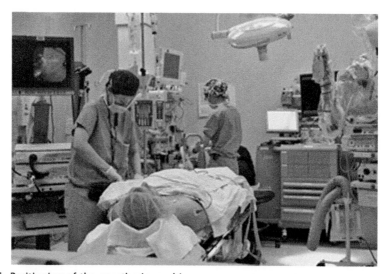

Fig. 6. Positioning of the anesthesia machine.

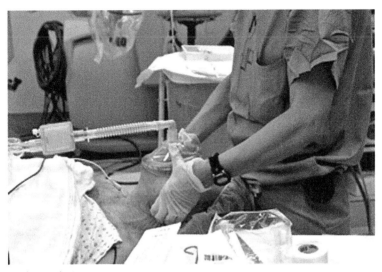

Fig. 7. Mask ventilation.

intubation. Following intubation, neuromuscular blockade is instituted to allow for sufficient muscular flaccidity to place the mouth gag and to eliminate movement in the field when electrocautery is applied to pharyngeal muscles. We typically use infusions of cisatracurium, typically at 1.5 μg/kg/min, but a single bolus of vecuronium or rocuronium may be sufficient for short cases.

POSTOPERATIVE PERIOD

The availability of otolaryngologists, anesthesiologists, and nurses who can assess and manage the TORS patient in the postoperative period greatly influences postoperative airway management. Although intubation for one and a half days during the postoperative period would obviate the need for airway evaluation and management, the morbidity of prolonged intubation cannot be discounted. In O'Malley and Weinstein's seminal report on 27 TORS patients, most of the patients were intubated postoperatively for 24 to 72 hours.[7] In Iseli and colleagues'[20] report of 54 TORS patients, 12 patients remained intubated postoperatively for 48 hours and 2 patients had a tracheotomy performed at the time of TORS. In Moore and colleagues'[13] report of 45 TORS patients, 14 patients (all with base of tongue lesions) had a tracheotomy performed at the time of TORS. The benefits of immediate postoperative extubation are self-evident; however, the need for a safe and adequate airway is paramount. The present approach at the University of Pennsylvania is to leave all patients intubated (1) when the dissection is adjacent to the vallecula or epiglottis so postoperative swelling will be suspected, (2) in a prolonged case in which tongue swelling is expected, and (3) during most TORS supraglottic partial laryngectomies. Our indications for a tracheostomy are in (1) any resection that involves both the tongue base and a portion of the epiglottis, (2) any patient in whom postoperative emergency intubation is expected to be difficult (ie, prior radiation), or (3) a patient with a medical indication (ie, morbid obesity). All patients are given dexamethasone 10 mg at the outset of the case and 6 mg every 6 hours until hospital discharge. Patients are discharged with a medrol dose pack.

TORS-related postoperative complications are relatively rare occurrences. In O'Malley and Weinstein's[7] radical tonsillectomy series, 2 patients experienced moderate trismus, 1 patient required a tracheotomy for exacerbation of obstructive sleep apnea following TORS, and 1 patient experienced significant bleeding. In Iseli and colleagues'[20] series, 3 patients required an unplanned tracheotomy, and 3 patients experienced significant bleeding. Genden and colleagues[11] reported no complications in a series of 18 TORS patients. The early postoperative complication rates for TORS appear comparable with the complication rates for the alternative therapies of nonrobotic transoral surgery, open surgery, and concurrent chemotherapy with radiation therapy.[14,21]

TREATMENT AFTER TORS

After TORS and pathology review, the patient is counseled on the need for further surgical and medical treatment. When oncologically indicated, a staged neck dissection(s) is performed 1 to 3 weeks following TORS. At the authors' institution, the neck dissection is performed after TORS to avoid the creation of a communication between the pharynx and neck. Additionally, performing the neck dissection as a separate procedure allows for shorter operative time and decreased tissue manipulation, minimizing laryngopharyngeal swelling that may result in the need for a tracheostomy. Other reports advocate neck dissection at the time of TORS, citing concerns of delay in adjuvant therapy and prolonging the overall treatment duration.[11,13,20] Adjuvant therapies following TORS include chemotherapy, radiation therapy, or concurrent chemotherapy and radiation therapy. Considerations for adjuvant therapy include tumor size, extracapsular spread, and histopathologic characteristics suggestive of a poor prognosis. The determination for adjuvant therapies should be made in conjunction with a head and neck cancer tumor board composed of otolaryngologists, medical oncologists, radiation oncologists, pathologists, and neuroradiologists.

FUTURE APPLICATIONS FOR ROBOTIC SURGERY IN THE HEAD AND NECK

The FDA approval of TORS has opened the gateway for other clinical applications of robotic surgery in the head and neck. Reports evaluating the applications of TORS in sleep surgery,[22] skull base surgery,[23–25] pediatric airway surgery,[26] and free flap reconstruction[27,28] may be a harbinger of the vast potential for TORS. Recent studies have also suggested that robot-assisted thyroid surgery may be an alternative treatment option to traditional open thyroid surgery.[29,30] As robotic surgery in the head and neck continues to enter the surgical mainstream, questions regarding feasibility, safety, cost-effectiveness, and patient outcomes will only increase.[31] Furthermore, the demand for physicians and health care providers who can care for these patients will also steadily grow. Further studies of long-term oncologic outcomes, cost, and quality of life are warranted.

SUMMARY

In the current information-rich consumer-focused health care environment, greater numbers of well-informed patients are seeking out TORS exclusively because of its minimally invasive approach. Individuals who need to avoid the morbidity of a larger surgery because of comorbid medical disease, as well as patients whose personal desires or professional obligations will not allow them to suffer a prolonged postoperative recovery or significant changes in voice or appearance can take advantage of the potential benefits of TORS. TORS allows exceptional surgical treatment of head and neck disease while minimizing morbidity and improving functional outcome as compared with open surgical approaches.

REFERENCES

1. Hockstein NG, Nolan JP, O'Malley BW Jr, et al. Robotic microlaryngeal surgery: a technical feasibility study using the daVinci surgical robot and an airway mannequin. Laryngoscope 2005;115:780.
2. Hockstein NG, Nolan JP, O'Malley BW Jr, et al. Robot-assisted pharyngeal and laryngeal microsurgery: results of robotic cadaver dissections. Laryngoscope 2005;115:1003.
3. Weinstein GS, O'Malley BW Jr, Hockstein NG. Transoral robotic surgery: supraglottic laryngectomy in a canine model. Laryngoscope 2005;115:1315.
4. O'Malley BW, Weinstein GS, Hockstein NG. Transoral robotic surgery (TORS): glottic microsurgery in a canine model. J Voice 2006;20:263–8.
5. Hockstein NG, O'Malley BW Jr, Weinstein GS. Assessment of intraoperative safety in transoral robotic surgery. Laryngoscope 2006;116:165.
6. O'Malley BW Jr, Weinstein GS, Snyder W, et al. Transoral robotic surgery (TORS) for base of tongue neoplasms. Laryngoscope 2006;116:1465.
7. Weinstein GS, O'Malley BW Jr, Snyder W, et al. Transoral robotic surgery: radical tonsillectomy. Arch Otolaryngol Head Neck Surg 2007;133:1220.
8. Haus BM, Kambham N, Le D, et al. Surgical robotic applications in otolaryngology. Laryngoscope 2003;113:1139.
9. Solares CA, Strome M. Transoral robot-assisted CO2 laser supraglottic laryngectomy: experimental and clinical data. Laryngoscope 2007;117:817.
10. Desai SC, Sung CK, Jang DW, et al. Transoral robotic surgery using a carbon dioxide flexible laser for tumors of the upper aerodigestive tract. Laryngoscope 2008;118:2187.
11. Genden EM, Desai S, Sung CK. Transoral robotic surgery for the management of head and neck cancer: a preliminary experience. Head Neck 2009;31:283.
12. Weinstein GS, O'Malley BW Jr, Snyder W, et al. Transoral robotic surgery: supraglottic partial laryngectomy. Ann Otol Rhinol Laryngol 2007;116:19.
13. Moore EJ, Olsen KD, Kasperbauer JL. Transoral robotic surgery for oropharyngeal squamous cell carcinoma: a prospective study of feasibility and functional outcomes. Laryngoscope 2009;119(11):2156–64.
14. Holsinger FC, McWhorter AJ, Ménard M, et al. Transoral lateral oropharyngectomy for squamous cell carcinoma of the tonsillar region: I. Technique, complications, and functional results. Arch Otolaryngol Head Neck Surg 2005;131:583.
15. Rudert HH, Werner JA, Höft S. Transoral carbon dioxide laser resection of supraglottic carcinoma. Ann Otol Rhinol Laryngol 1999;108:819.
16. Mandel JE, Weller GE, Chennupati SK, et al. Transglottic high frequency jet ventilation for management of laryngeal fracture associated with air bag deployment injury. J Clin Anesth 2008;20:369–71.
17. Higgs A, Clark E, Premraj K. Low-skill fibreoptic intubation: use of the Aintree Catheter with the classic LMA. Anaesthesia 2005;60:915–20.
18. Lange M, Frommer M, Redel A, et al. Comparison of the Glidescope and Airtraq optical laryngoscopes in patients undergoing direct microlaryngoscopy. Anaesthesia 2009;64:323–8.
19. Racine SX, Solis A, Hamou NA, et al. Face mask ventilation in edentulous patients: a comparison of mandibular groove and lower lip placement. Anesthesiology 2010;112:1190.
20. Iseli TA, Kulbersh BD, Iseli CE, et al. Functional outcomes after transoral robotic surgery for head and neck cancer. Otolaryngol Head Neck Surg 2009;141:166.

21. Machtay M, Rosenthal DI, Hershock D, et al. Organ preservation therapy using induction plus concurrent chemoradiation for advanced resectable oropharyngeal carcinoma: a University of Pennsylvania Phase II Trial. J Clin Oncol 2002; 20:3964–71.
22. Vicini C, Dallan I, Canzi P, et al. Transoral robotic tongue base resection in obstructive sleep apnoea-hypopnoea syndrome: a preliminary report. ORL J Otorhinolaryngol Relat Spec 2010;72:22.
23. Lee JY, O'Malley BW, Newman JG, et al. Transoral robotic surgery of craniocervical junction and atlantoaxial spine: a cadaveric study. J Neurosurg Spine 2010;12:13.
24. O'Malley BW Jr, Weinstein GS. Robotic skull base surgery: preclinical investigations to human clinical application. Arch Otolaryngol Head Neck Surg 2007;133: 1215.
25. O'Malley BW Jr, Weinstein GS. Robotic anterior and midline skull base surgery: preclinical investigations. Int J Radiat Oncol Biol Phys 2007;69:S125.
26. Rahbar R, Ferrari LR, Borer JG, et al. Robotic surgery in the pediatric airway: application and safety. Arch Otolaryngol Head Neck Surg 2007;133:46.
27. Mukhija VK, Sung CK, Desai SC, et al. Transoral robotic assisted free flap reconstruction. Otolaryngol Head Neck Surg 2009;140:124.
28. Selber JC, Robb G, Serletti JM, et al. Transoral robotic free flap reconstruction of oropharyngeal defects: a preclinical investigation. Plast Reconstr Surg 2010; 125:896.
29. Kang SW, Lee SC, Lee SH, et al. Robotic thyroid surgery using a gasless, transaxillary approach and the da Vinci S system: the operative outcomes of 338 consecutive patients. Surgery 2009;146(6):1048–55.
30. Kang SW, Jeong JJ, Yun JS, et al. Robot-assisted endoscopic surgery for thyroid cancer: experience with the first 100 patients. Surg Endosc 2009;23(11): 2399–406.
31. Weinstein GS, O'Malley BW Jr, Desai SC, et al. Transoral robotic surgery: does the ends justify the means? Curr Opin Otolaryngol Head Neck Surg 2009; 17(2):126–31.

Electromyographic (EMG) Neuromonitoring in Otolaryngology-Head and Neck Surgery

Francis X. Dillon, MD[a,b,*]

KEYWORDS

- Head and neck surgery • Electromyography
- Recurrent laryngeal nerve injury • Phrenic nerve injury
- Vocal cord paralysis • Intraoperative nerve monitoring
- NIM tube • Neck dissection

Intraoperative neuromonitoring (IONM) is a relatively recent advance in electromyography (EMG) applied to otolaryngology–head and neck surgery. Its purpose is to allow real-time identification and functional assessment of vulnerable nerves during surgery. The nerves most often monitored in head and neck surgery are the motor branch of the facial nerve (VII), the recurrent or inferior laryngeal nerves (X), the vagus nerve (X), and the spinal accessory nerve (XI), with other cranial lower nerves monitored less frequently. Morbidity from trauma to these nerves is significant and obvious, such as unilateral facial paresis. Although functional restorative surgery is usually considered to repair the effects of such an insult, the importance of preventing nerve injury in head and neck surgery is obvious.

The goal in providing anesthesia during these procedures is to allow adequate depth of anesthesia while accomplishing neuromonitoring. Although the use of IONM is common in middle ear and parotid surgeries in which the facial (VII) nerve is at risk of injury, the recent advent of endotracheal tubes with embedded electrodes, such as the nerve integrity monitor (NIM) tube (Xomed, Jacksonville, FL, USA) or of disposable electrodes applied to standard endotracheal tubes (eg, Dragonfly Stick-on Electrode, IOM Products, Inc, Ventura, CA, USA)[1,2] to monitor recurrent laryngeal nerve function intraoperatively provides another degree of safety for patients undergoing thyroid and other neck surgeries. The standardization of protocols for neuromonitoring in

[a] Department of Anesthesia, Massachusetts Eye and Ear Infirmary, 243 Charles Street, Room 712, Boston, MA 02114, USA
[b] Department of Anaesthesia, Harvard Medical School, Boston, MA, USA
* Department of Anesthesia, Massachusetts Eye and Ear Infirmary, 243 Charles Street, Room 712, Boston, MA 02114.
E-mail address: francis_dillon@meei.harvard.edu

Anesthesiology Clin 28 (2010) 423–442
doi:10.1016/j.anclin.2010.07.011
1932-2275/10/$ – see front matter © 2010 Published by Elsevier Inc.

head and neck surgery is an area of great interest[3,4] and will contribute greatly to patient safety and the quality of research in the field of intraoperative nerve preservation.

SCOPE AND DEFINITIONS

This article focuses on the anesthetic considerations pertinent to IONM of peripheral cranial nerves during otolaryngologic–head and neck surgery. The specific modality of IONM is EMG, both spontaneous and evoked. Spontaneous and evoked EMGs are "cousins" to a modality anesthesiologists commonly use while administering routine anesthetics: neuromuscular junction (NMJ) monitoring. Spontaneous EMG monitors the spontaneous electrical activity of muscle cells, and had its initial application in diagnosing neurologic illnesses and traumatic denervations, in which pathologic muscle electrical activity was found to be distinct from normal. With evoked EMG, the nerve innervating a muscle is stimulated with a voltage and current that is somewhat supraphysiologic (of the order of 0.5 mA), and the purpose is not neurodiagnosis but spatial identification of nerves to preserve them from injury, usually during operations.

In comparison, NMJ monitoring is most accurately termed *mechanomyography* of the motor division of nerves, such as the ulnar nerve, after electrical stimulus with gel-surface electrodes. IONM, however, is more accurately termed *spontaneous* or *evoked EMG*. EMG implies that the finer aspects of the wave impulse (spontaneous or evoked) may be examined with an oscillographic cathode ray tube or, currently, with signal-processing hardware and software based in a small computer.

The commonly used peripherals, or data inputting devices, used in IONM are stimulating electrodes shaped like probes, needles, or surgical instruments; they may even be specially designed and insulated surgical instruments such as drills that are used to stimulate nerves and muscles during dissection. Several kinds of recording electrodes are also available; needle electrodes placed in target muscles are the most commonly used. Their wires or leads connect to the recording hardware. More recently, a specially designed tracheal tube with embedded wire surface electrodes (eg, NIM tube, Xomed, Jacksonville, FL, USA) has been used for the dedicated task of monitoring spontaneous and evoked potentials of the vocalis muscle. This device, the NIM tube, and other similar devices made by other manufacturers, are used intraoperatively to monitor the function of the vocalis muscle and the nerves which innervate it, that is, the recurrent laryngeal nerve, and more proximally, the vagus nerve.

Why choose EMG over mechanomyography? Mechanomyography is a simple, noninvasive, and inexpensive means of monitoring the NMJ and, specifically, titrating the neuromuscular blockade: It allows physicians to easily visualize the "train of four" and semiquantitatively estimate the percentage of neuromuscular blockade present. For example, one twitch means 90% blockade, according to the convention. Electromyography, however, allows physicians to visualize the motor action potential as a waveform. It is more sensitive and may be stored and analyzed as data. However, the essential stimulus and response are the same for EMG and mechanomyography.

HISTORY

The first attempt at sparing the facial nerve during parotid surgery was recorded by Thomas Carwardine in 1907.[5,6] He used careful dissection to identify numerous branches of the facial nerve in his patients, and although palsies were common after surgery, these were not permanent or significant in most patients.

Similarly, in early otolaryngologic practice in the 1940s and 1950s, sound anatomic knowledge,[7–10] experience, and especially visual identification of the cranial nerves in the surgical field were established[11] as the gold standard of facial and recurrent laryngeal nerve preservation during surgery. Authors still reinforce this approach, pointing out that EMG and other modalities for IONM are merely adjuncts to careful visual identification and preservation of the nerve.

Before EMG was developed, trained surgical assistants would watch the anesthetized patient's target muscles (eg, the *orbicularis oculi*) during middle ear or parotid surgery. Any mechanical stimulus such as stretching or dissecting near the nerve would cause twitching of the muscle and alert the surgeon to impending trauma. As a first step it was useful, though not particularly sensitive or specific. For example, mechanical retraction of the nerve would not pinpoint exactly where a nerve or branch of one was, a nerve could not be reproducibly stimulated using traction or mechanical stimulus without risking trauma to the nerve.

Feinstein[12] first mentioned the use of EMG for diagnosing disorders of the facial and recurrent laryngeal nerves (nonoperatively) in 1946, whereas Cawthorne[13–14] was the first to use intraoperative electrical stimulation of the facial nerve. He and his assistants witnessed visually or through palpation the resulting muscle movements in the surgical field. The first use of EMG to identify the facial nerve intraoperatively was reported by Delgado and colleagues in 1979,[15] and Brennan and colleagues[16] published their account of investigations of recurrent laryngeal nerve monitoring in 2001. The use of this modality became common in acoustic neuroma, mastoidectomy, and other surgeries during which the facial nerve is at risk of injury. In the 1990s, IONM of the recurrent laryngeal nerve became more common, and now is routine, especially for surgeons more recently out of training or those whose practices specialize in thyroid or other surgeries posing a risk to the vagus, recurrent laryngeal, and other lower cranial nerves.[4]

EMG began as an experimental diagnostic technique in the 1940s to the 1960s,[17] but it did not become incorporated in surgical practice until the late 1970s and 1980s, when it was used with evoked responses (ie, brief pulses of current of 1 ms or less and 0.05 mA at 1 Hz) as a means of identifying nerves in the operative field. Spontaneous EMG allowed visualization of spontaneous muscle action potentials (MAPs) from nerves with tonic or "background" activity, and also from mechanical stimuli such as dissection or retraction. Evoked EMG lent another degree of sensitivity to the process of intraoperative neuroprotection because it allowed the use of the repeated supraphysiologic stimuli to identify the innervated muscle in the surgical field as an adjunct to nerve visualization. IONM became useful in identifying and mapping nerves and branches, especially during parotidectomy. Reducing the current of the stimuli in evoked EMG also allowed the nerve's functional status to be determined. An injured nerve required a higher stimulus threshold than an intact one, allowing early or subtle injury to be identified.

More recently, incorporation of cathode ray oscillograph tubes,[9,13] and later, personal computers and peripherals for storage and analysis of waveforms, made IONM data reproducible and reliable. Many technicians (usually audiologists) became experienced in intraoperative setup and the gathering and interpretation of data. The last step in this progression is occurring now: the incorporation of international consensus standards and protocols to make the information obtained from IONM specific, diagnostic, and sensitive.

Nerves commonly monitored during otolaryngology–head and neck surgery are (1) the superior laryngeal, recurrent laryngeal, and vagus nerves during thyroidectomy, parathyroidectomy, neck dissection, carotid endarterectomy, and other surgeries in the anterior cervical region; (2) the motor branch of the facial nerve during tympanic, mastoid, parotid, and other otologic surgeries; (3) other cranial or cervical spinal nerves and branches during neck dissection; and (4) the lower cranial or cervical spinal nerve during lateral skull base surgery. Specific aspects of these techniques and their relevance to otolaryngologic anesthesia are summarized.

GENERAL ANESTHETIC CONSIDERATIONS FOR ALL IONM AND EMG PROCEDURES USED IN OTOLARYNGOLOGIC SURGERY

Which anesthetic technique is compatible with the type of monitoring used in a given procedure? Several modalities are available for monitoring the central and peripheral nervous system during otolaryngologic and neurotologic surgery. **Tables 1** and **2** list the conventional types of monitoring and the anesthetic agents that affect or have no effect on the specific type of monitoring. For the sake of comparison, other modalities besides IONM (spontaneous and evoked EMG) are included in **Tables 1** and **2**, although they are not topics of review in this article.

The use of a total intravenous technique, consisting of a short-acting narcotic through infusion combined with propofol, is generally considered compatible with all types of IONM. Likewise, the use of nitrous oxide and volatile agents is acceptable. The main drug categories to be avoided in IONM are the neuromuscular blocking agents and local anesthetics, and the inability to use them makes the anesthetic more of a challenge. The neuromuscular blocking drugs may be used at induction and intubation provided their effects have cleared by the time IONM begins. Therefore, either succinylcholine (1–2 mg/kg) or rocuronium (0.5 mg/kg) are suitable drugs for intubation.

VAGUS AND RECURRENT LARYNGEAL NERVE MONITORING DURING THYROIDECTOMY, PARATHYROIDECTOMY, AND OTHER ANTERIOR CERVICAL SURGERY

As remotely as 1938,[18,19] and as recently as the present time,[4,9] authors have advocated visual identification of the recurrent[20] and superior[21] laryngeal nerves during thyroidectomy and other surgeries as a means of avoiding trauma. Riddell[10] actually tested (and proved) the hypothesis of visual identification being superior to nonidentification of the recurrent laryngeal nerve as a way to protect it during thyroidectomy. Both visual identification and IONM seem to be a safe and reliable means of avoiding trauma to the nerve[21]; an extraordinarily large study may be necessary to show the superiority of IONM.[22] In a historical cohort study involving 1450 nerves at risk, Cavicchi and colleagues[23] showed that neither visual identification nor IONM is inferior. Clearly the traditional emphasis on anatomic knowledge and visual identification through careful dissection is supported by this and several older studies.

The debate about the superiority of IONM to visual identification is ongoing.[1–5,20–30] Perhaps it is fairer to say that use of the two methods is an attempt to improve the quality and safety of nerve preservation during otolaryngologic–head and neck surgery. When thyroidectomy was undertaken before concerted efforts were made to identify the recurrent laryngeal nerve, perhaps one in eight nerves were injured afterward. Today, the standard of safety has increased tremendously, to only a percent or so of postoperative nerve injury. Authors in the field believe there is still considerable room for improvement. Certainly when less-invasive techniques of thyroid surgery, such as robotic-assisted endoscopic surgery,[31] are more widely adopted, IONM will probably be used to help improve the safety of these procedures also.

The vagus (X) and its branches (**Fig. 1**) are the nerves most frequently monitored during thyroidectomy, parathyroidectomy, neck dissection, carotid endarterectomy, and skull base surgery. The vagus's branch to the intrinsic laryngeal muscles (ie, the recurrent laryngeal nerve) is the one most at risk during thyroidectomy. The superior laryngeal nerve, another branch of X, is of less consequence to the voice and glottic function because it innervates only one muscle in the larynx, the cricothyroid muscle. The superior laryngeal nerve may be,[26] but is not usually, monitored during head and neck surgeries.

ANESTHETIC CONSIDERATIONS FOR NIM TUBE MONITORING DURING THYROID SURGERY

Anesthesiologists are usually asked to tailor their technique to allow for efficient placement and accurate positioning of the NIM tube (**Fig. 2**). Ideally, the surgeon and anesthesiologist will confer at length about the placement and use of the NIM tube.

The overall goals are to (1) provide for a quick induction, intubation, and positioning, including neck extension; (2) allow partial emergence or lightening immediately after intubation so that respiratory variation in the vocalis muscle (ie, accurate tube placement with good electrical contact) may be demonstrated; then (3) quickly deepen the patient with intravenous anesthetic such as propofol to prevent any movement of the tube from coughing.

An alternative approach to the use of the specialized NIM tube or applied electrodes[2] involves continuous intraoperative observation of vocal cord movement using laryngeal mask airway (LMA) and fiberoptic bronchoscope. With this approach, which is discussed in the article by Mandel elsewhere in this issue, movement of the vocal cords after electrical stimulation of the recurrent laryngeal or vagal nerves is documented with videography by way of fiberoptic endoscope.

After induction, lightening or partial emergence from the induction dose, and optimal placement of the NIM tube, the patient must be maintained at a certain depth of anesthesia. It must be deep enough to assure that no spontaneous EMG activity occurs in the vocalis muscles, but not too deep to prevent hypotension or delayed emergence. The audiologist will ordinarily be able to monitor the tonic EMG in the resting vocalis muscle and determine, usually before coughing occurs, that the patient is getting light from the induction dose.

The induction and intubation sequence, if performed properly, will save time and allow for accurate readings and good quality of data from the monitoring equipment. Induction agents ideally should clear rapidly and the patient should lighten to the extent that spontaneous vocalis muscle EMG activity may be observed from the two electrodes of the NIM tube. Once the placement of the tube is deemed optimal (through the presence of good bilateral impedance readings and spontaneous respiratory variation from the tonic activity of the vocalis muscle), then the patient is deepened, skin is prepared, and the operation begins.

The authors' specific induction sequence is as follows:

1. Preinduction medication with remifentanil, 0.5 mcg/kg, midazolam, 0.01 to 0.025 mg/kg, and rocuronium, 0.04 mg/kg, plus glycopyrrolate, 0.002 mg/kg (to attenuate airway secretions)
2. Induction with propofol, 2 to 3 mg/kg, and succinylcholine, 2 mg/kg
3. Intubation with a dry styletted NIM tube of the largest practical size possible (see later discussion) to allow for good contact between the electrodes and the tracheal mucosa
4. Inhalation of a 1.0% fraction of inspired isoflurane or other similar fractions of other volatile anesthetic agents, with or without nitrous oxide
5. Extension of the neck with the thyroid bag, foam pillow, or folded sheet, to position the patient for surgery

Table 1
Types of intraoperative neurophysiologic monitoring and the effects of various anesthetic drugs on them

Type or Modality of Neurophysiologic Monitoring	Surgery Examples	Region	Volatile Agents (eg, Isoflurane)	Neuromuscular Blocking Agents	Total Intravenous Anesthesia		Local Anesthetics	Nitrous Oxide
					Opioids	Propofol		
Brainstem auditory evoked response	Acoustic neuroma, trigeminal neuralgia, facial nerve decompression, endolymphatic sac	Cerebellopontine angle, mastoid region, middle ear	1	0	0	1	0	0
Cortical somatosensory evoked potentials	Spinal fusion, tumor, decompression	Spine (posterior columns)	2 (affect amplitude and latency of waveforms)	0	0	0	2	1 Nitrous oxide (affects amplitude only)
Neuromuscular junction monitoring	Neuromuscular blockade in anesthesia	Ulnar nerve, facial nerve, posterior tibial nerve	0	2	0	0	2	0
IONM: spontaneous EMG	Thyroid, parathyroid, parotid, neck dissection, skull base	Facial, vagal, recurrent laryngeal, other crania l nerves	0	2	0	0	2	0

IONM: evoked EMG								
IONM: evoked EMG	Thyroid, parathyroid, parotid, neck dissection, skull base	Facial, vagal, recurrent laryngeal, other crania I nerves.	0	2	0	0	2	0
MEP	Spinal fusion, tumor, decompression	Spine (anterior columns)	2	2	0	0	2	0
EEG (BIS)	All	All	2	0	2	2	0	1
EEG	Carotid endarterectomy	Carotid	2	0	2	2	2	2

Scale: 0 = insensitive; 1 = somewhat sensitive; 2 = very sensitive.

The two classes of drug to be avoided during monitoring of facial, recurrent laryngeal, vagal, and other cranial motor nerves are neuromuscular blocking agents and local anesthetics. Both may increase latency, decrease amplitude, and increase stimulus threshold of the evoked response, or may decrease the sensitivity of EMG to nerve injury.

A conventional balanced anesthetic (opioid, nitrous oxide/oxygen, volatile agent) is suitable for surgery using EMG and EEMG.

Abbreviations: BIS, bispectral electroencephalogram; EEG, electroencephalogram; EMG, electromyogram; IONM, intraoperative nerve monitoring; MEP, motor evoked potentials.

Data from Johnson S, Goldenberg D. Intraoperative monitoring of the recurrent laryngeal nerve during revision thyroid surgery. Otolaryngol Clin North Am 2008;41(6):1147–54.

Table 2
Effects of certain agents on electromyographic and brainstem auditory evoked response intraoperative monitoring during otolaryngologic surgery[a]

Agent	Effect
Local anesthetics (lidocaine, bupivacaine, cocaine, tetracaine)	Altered latency and amplitude of CMAP after impaired propagation of potentials
Neuromuscular blockade (succinylcholine, atracurium, mivacurium, vecuronium, pancuronium, doxacurium, pipecuronium)	Spontaneous and triggered EMG abolished until worn off or reversed (can be lengthy period)
Local or systemic hypothermia, cold irrigation fluid	BAER absolute, interpeak latencies prolonged, wave amplitudes diminish, neurotonic stimulation of EMG activity
Tissue compression, retraction	BAER averaged auditory responses degraded or abolished, EMG amplitudes and latency affected
Inadequate ventilation, hemodilution, systemic hypotension, regional ischemia	BAER reduced oxygen affects endocochlear potentials, decreases cochlear output

Abbreviations: BAER, brainstem auditory evoked response; CMAP, compound muscle action potential; EMG, electromyogram.
  [a] Facial nerve (VII), vagus nerve (X), superior laryngeal (X), and recurrent laryngeal (X) nerves.
  Data from Edwards BM, Kileny PR. Intraoperative monitoring of cranial nerves. In: Canalis RF, Lambert PR, editors. The ear: comprehensive otology. Philadelphia: Lippincott Williams & Wilkins; 2000. p. 284.

6. In less than 5 minutes, anesthesia should lighten to the extent that respiratory variation and spontaneous recurrent laryngeal nerve activity may be observed by the audiologist, surgeon, or anesthesiologist monitoring the NIM
7. Immediately, to avoid the risk of coughing and tube displacement, another 0.25 to 1 mg/kg propofol is given intravenously and the inspired concentration of volatile agent is simultaneously increased
8. The tube may be taped in place and supported with a metal frame as usual
9. Eye tape or lubricant may be applied.

A few more details about insertion and positioning of the NIM tube are important. According to the manufacturer (Xomed, Jacksonville, FL, USA), the tube should be inserted with a stylet, preferably under direct visualization, with the use of a water-based, nonanesthetic lubricant. (Note that the position statement of Randolph and Dralle[4] contradicts this and insists that no lubricant should be used.) The use of a tube slightly larger than normal is advocated by the manufacturer and other authors, because the surface electrodes of the tube will then be in better contact with the vocal cords. For most women and men, this typically involves a 7.0-mm or 8.0-mm internal diameter (ID) NIM tube, respectively. Good contact assures good initial respiratory variation and good symmetric impedance readings from either vocalis electrode. If these two conditions are met, the tube likely will have been optimally placed and evoked responses will be of good amplitude.

Although the use of either succinylcholine or a short-acting nondepolarizing neuromuscular blocking drug such as rocuronium is common, some practitioners prefer to avoid neuromuscular blockade altogether. They intubate under deep total intravenous anesthesia, perhaps supplemented with a volatile anesthetic. In these cases, the use of topical laryngotracheal anesthesia (LTA) using 4% lidocaine is helpful for blunting the stimulus of intubation. However, this practice is not recommended in the NIM tube package insert.

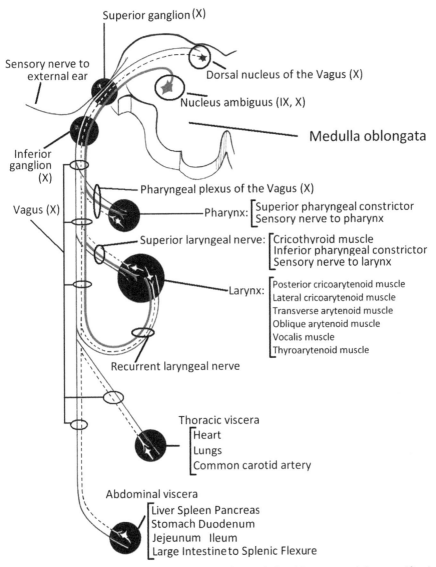

Fig. 1. The vagus (cranial nerve X) originates in the medulla oblongata and then ramifies in the superior and inferior vagal ganglia in the neck. Its first major branch is the pharyngeal plexus of the vagus. Its next branch is the recurrent laryngeal nerve, which innervates the intrinsic muscles of the larynx responsible for phonation and glottis opening. Inferior to this it wanders (hence the name *vagus*) through the thoracic and abdominal viscera, innervating them with autonomic motor and sensory nerve fibers.

To facilitate accurate placement, the NIM tube has an embedded blue dye stripe (or lettering stripe) oriented anteriorly (12 o'clock) along the shaft of the tube. Located at 9 o'clock (left) and 3 o'clock (right) are the embedded wire electrodes contacting the vocal cords and underlying vocalis muscles. The tube placement itself is critical because small displacements (rotation or insertion/removal) can cause large changes in impedance and evoked responses. The tube depth of insertion is very important,

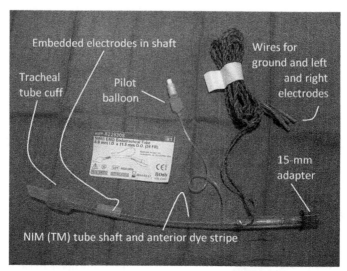

Fig. 2. The nerve integrity monitor (NIM) tube, manufactured by Xomed, Jacksonville, FL, USA. This device is one of the most commonly used for intraoperative nerve monitoring of the vagus and recurrent laryngeal nerves. It records two channels, one each an embedded electrode that is in contact with the vocalis muscles, left and right. A blue orientation stripe is embedded in the anterior direction to allow accurate placement. The tube is inserted, styletted, with a conventional oral laryngoscope or fiberoptic bronchoscope, or a GlideScope device.

because the embedded electrodes are of finite length and must be apposed to the vocal cords for optimal readings. In an Asian population, Lu and colleagues[1] showed that depth of NIM tube insertion was consistent in men and women. They intubated 105 patients undergoing thyroid surgery with a Xomed NIM tube, using conventional laryngoscopy and direct visualization. Of these patients, 99 (94.3%) had successful IONM with the initial endotracheal tube position, and 6 (5.7%) needed further tube depth adjustment with fiber-optic bronchoscopy. All patients ultimately had successful monitoring. The investigators found that the optimal mean tube depth measured from the teeth was 20.6 ± 0.97 cm in men and 19.6 ± 1.0 cm in women ($P \leq .01$). Taller subjects had a trend toward deeper tube depth ($P \leq .05$). This benchmark of tube depth of course may vary with other patient populations. They concluded that the mean depth of the NIM EMG tube is a useful reference value for detecting the malposition of electrodes and adjusting the depth of tube during thyroid surgery. During these intraoperative manipulations, the anesthesiologist will usually be asked to insert or remove the tube by a centimeter or so to return it to its original place. Putting an indelible ink mark or a piece of tape as an indicator is helpful to allow the tube to be replaced at its original location.

After induction and intubation, and before incision, or intraoperatively, these position adjustments may be made to optimize otherwise unsatisfactory baseline readings. These adjustments may be performed with plain visualization of the face and tracheal tube using conventional laryngoscopy, fiber-optic laryngoscopy, or GlideScope laryngoscopy. The GlideScope is becoming widely used for precise insertion and manipulation of the embedded electrode or tubes with adhesive electrodes. The advantage of the GlideScope is that the surgeon may use the device to assist and confirm placement of the tube, which expedites the procedure because correct initial placement usually avoids the need for further manipulation.

After this process the tube is securely taped. The tube may move during surgery for at least four reasons: (1) blunt and sharp dissection and retraction involves manipulating the larynx and, indirectly, the tube, (2) stimulating the recurrent laryngeal nerve causes adduction of the cords and small displacements result, (3) some surgeons, as a means of showing nerve integrity, stimulate the recurrent laryngeal nerve and simultaneously palpate for vocal cord adduction, and (4) patient movement may occur because muscle relaxation is contraindicated and anesthetic depth may not be excessive.

A learning curve[32] is clear when using the NIM tube; namely, the percentage of tubes placed rapidly and the number of good readings increase with the number of tubes inserted. Dralle[30] noted that as the cumulative number of NIM tubes placed totaled first 50, then 100, then 150, the percentage of tubes placed rapidly and accurately increased from 80% to 92% to 98% ($P \leq .05$ for the trend). This trend represents a very high standard of expertise for placing the tubes.

The goal in maintenance, given good tube placement at the outset, is to keep an adequate depth of anesthesia to blunt the spontaneous EMG activity of the vocalis muscles. That is, no respiratory variation or spontaneous MAPs should be seen. If they are, the custom at the authors' institution is for the audiologist to immediately notify the anesthesiologist. Respiratory variation in the EMG indicates a lighter-than-desirable intraoperative plane of anesthesia. Deepening of anesthesia is usually necessary, either through increasing the inspired concentration of volatile agent or giving additional propofol (0.25–1.00 mg/kg intravenously), or both. The goal is timely deepening to avoid coughing on and displacement of the tube.

Furthermore, a plan must be in place to deal with intraoperative loss of signal after initial successful NIM tube placement. Randolph and Dralle[4] proposed an algorithm that first involves a definition of loss of signal being either change from initial satisfactory EMG; no signal or quantitatively low EMG response (ie, ≤ 100 μV) with stimulation using a stimulus of 1 to 2 mA, and with dry surgical field conditions; or no laryngeal twitch or observed glottic twitch visualized. If signal is lost, the surgeon will attempt to troubleshoot it by first seeing if the problem is in the stimulus or recording part of the apparatus.

If a palpable laryngeal twitch occurs during stimulus but no visible or strong signal is present, then endotracheal tube malposition is a strong possibility, as is a fault elsewhere in the recording part. Therefore, while the anesthesiologist suctions the airway and inspects tube placement, the surgeon, audiologist, and others will check the recording part ground, interface box, and monitor connections, and assess the impedance of the wire/tracheal mucosa contacts. If these are satisfactory, the surgeon will stimulate the vagus (actually stimulating the recurrent laryngeal nerve upstream) while the anesthesiologist inserts, withdraws, or rotates the tube while the signal is observed. Lu and colleagues[1] found that insertion and withdrawal of the tube were needed almost equally as frequently, and rotation less frequently, to regain good signal strength. Usually this troubleshooting is successful.

If no palpable laryngeal twitch is present, then the crucial test is to directly stimulate a muscle in the operative field. If the muscle contracts, then the nonoperated side's vagus nerve is stimulated; if that yields a proper laryngeal evoked potential and twitch, then ipsilateral nerve injury should be considered. If the muscle does not contract in response to direct stimulation, then the stimulator, probe, stimulation side ground, interface box, monitor connections, operative field (eg, blood, secretions), and neuromuscular junction are assessed. Usually one of these will be found to be at fault.

Another patient safety issue in head and neck surgery is extension of the head and neck. Severe neck extension during anterior neck surgery has been reported to cause trauma to the brainstem or spinal cord, or hypoperfusion of the posterior circulation. Catastrophic quadriplegia or "locked in syndrome" has been reported after thyroid or anterior cervical disk surgery, although fortunately these are rare complications. Often the anesthesiologist and surgeon will both position the head and neck after induction and intubation to ensure that the occiput has adequate support and that the extension is not excessive. However, no readily available technology is in current use to monitor cord, brainstem, or brain functionality or perfusion during otolaryngology–head and neck surgery.

Fortunately the most common problem related to neck extension before or during surgery is movement of the embedded electrode tube. Extension of the neck will move the endotracheal tube relative to the carina and thus displace the electrodes from the optimal monitoring position.

Reverse Trendelenburg position is another potential risk factor for patient injury. Anesthetics of all classes are known to cause a robust sympatholysis, especially at induction. The sympatholysis has two aspects: decreased cardiac output and vasodilation. The vasodilation is mostly in the capacitance veins of the abdomen and legs, and the head-up table tilt (reverse Trendelenburg) or back-up tilt (semi-Fowler's) positions used in thyroid surgery potentiate this effect, often causing severe and recalcitrant hypotension. Even worse, propofol and other drugs used at induction obliterate the baroreceptor reflex. Physicians are advised to be prepared with glycopyrrolate, atropine, ephedrine, or phenylephrine to treat these effects. Infusions of phenylephrine during head and neck surgery may be needed throughout. Physicians should also beware of patients who are treated with angiotensin-converting enzyme inhibitors or angiotensin receptor blockers, because they may have recalcitrant hypotension from these drugs.[33] Is it possible that hypoperfusion of the nerve from Trendelenburg position and sympatholysis from anesthesia could cause a false-positive? Yes. In other words, abnormality in amplitude and latency could occur from ischemia and surgical trauma.

INTRAOPERATIVE MONITORING OF THE MOTOR BRANCH OF THE FACIAL NERVE DURING TYMPANIC, MASTOID, PAROTID, AND OTHER SURGERIES

The facial nerve is vulnerable to injury during many otolaryngologic procedures and parotidectomy rhytidectomy, and other head and neck procedures (**Fig. 3**). The typical IONM operation involving facial nerve monitoring, such as a tympanomastoidectomy, involves preoperative placement of facial nerve monitoring recording electrodes either awake or after induction and intubation. Surface gel or needle electrodes are placed in or overlying the orbicularis oculi and orbicularis oris muscles; these are the two positive channels most often monitored. A scalp electrode may be used for grounding the patient, or the ground may be placed elsewhere. The frontalis muscle may be monitored in addition to the standard two channels.

The stimulating electrode may be a monopolar or bipolar fine-tipped probe, or the electrode may be incorporated into surgical instruments like the rotary burr. Stimulating near the facial nerve will result in a characteristic waveform or audio signal. Based on the latency and amplitude of the waveform, the facial nerve may be identified and avoided during surgery. Typically the surgeon will demonstrate the intact nerve function several times: first as a means of localizing it, then during the procedure when the operative site is in proximity to it and the nerve is at special risk of injury, and lastly at the end of the procedure to show that the nerve is still functional from an EMG standpoint. Generally for facial nerve IONM, as in the case of the NIM tube, the monitor is a better negative predictor than a positive predictor of nerve injury, owing to the

DIAGRAM OF FACIAL NERVE ANATOMY

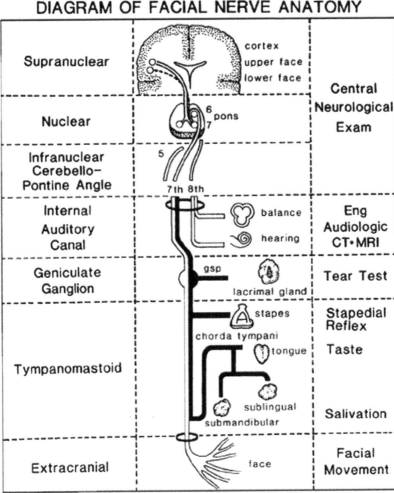

Fig. 3. Schematic of the facial nerve (cranial nerve VII). Note that from the level of the tympanomastoid region distally to the extracranial regions, the nerve is vulnerable during many common otolaryngologic procedures: myringotomy, tympanoplasty, mastoidectomy, parotidectomy, and rhytidectomy. (*Adapted from* May M. Anatomy for the clinician. In: May M, Schaitkin B, editors. The facial nerve. 2nd edition. New York: Thieme Medical Publishers, Inc; 2000. p. 19. Chapter 2; with permission.)

number of false-positives that may occur (eg, loss of grounding electrode; defective probe; current shunting from secretions, blood, or irrigant solution). In other words, if the nerve is still intact according to EMG assessment at the end of the procedure, then chances are very good that the nerve will be intact physiologically.

The parotid region is one in which the facial nerve is certainly at risk during dissection. In 1998, after reviewing the literature, Witt[34] suggested that the incidence of permanent facial nerve paralysis or paresis after surgery for benign parotid tumors was between 3% and 5%, and the incidence of postoperative transient facial nerve dysfunction was much higher, reportedly ranging from 8.2% to 65%. He noted the potentially catastrophic morbidity of corneal exposure leading to blindness, and therefore that transient facial nerve paresis, though not as morbid a complication as permanent paresis, was not an entirely benign complication.

ANESTHETIC CONSIDERATIONS DURING IONM OF THE MOTOR BRANCH OF THE FACIAL NERVE DURING TYMPANIC, MASTOID, PAROTID, AND OTHER SURGERIES

Patient movement is a primary concern, because of the use of powered surgical instruments and the proximity of the facial nerve to the operative site. As in anterior cervical surgery, valid concerns exist about the use of muscle relaxants and local anesthetics blocking the sensitivity of the IONM being used. Succinylcholine or rocuronium to facilitate intubation can be used initially but not afterward.

The microscopic field causes any blood loss during middle ear surgery to be problematic for surgeons, and even can make the surgery impossible. It complicates visualization and graft placement, among other things. Several methods to alter anesthetic technique are useful. A thorough review of these anesthesia considerations for middle ear surgery is provided by Irwin and Liang elsewhere in this issue.

As in thyroid, parathyroid, or other anterior neck surgery, the use of a short-acting opioid intravenous anesthetic such as remifentanil through infusion (0.01–0.25 µg/kg/min) will help deepen anesthesia and control blood pressure nicely. Anesthesiologists should discuss target mean or systolic pressures with the surgery team before starting, especially if the patient is hypertensive at baseline. These patients may not tolerate the lower cerebral perfusion pressures that normotensive patients might tolerate well.

Good blood pressure control implies good operating conditions but also may imply reduced cerebral perfusion pressure during otolaryngologic surgery. As in neck surgery, severe rotation and extension of the neck, coupled with low mean arterial pressures and mild reverse Trendelenburg (head-up) position, may predispose to worsening of hypotension. Readily available pressor (phenylephrine) through 100 µg boluses or infusion (0.1–0.5 µg/kg/min) is important; alternately, vasopressin infusion as a means of raising intraoperative blood pressure has been reported.[33] Invasive arterial pressure monitoring may help in a minority of instances but is not needed for most head and neck cases.

The use of nitrous oxide during middle ear surgeries, such as mastoidectomies and tympanoplasties, is somewhat controversial because of the implied risk of closed-space diffusion of air into a cavity containing nitrous oxide, or vice versa. Most authors allow for the use of nitrous oxide in craniotomy, tympanoplasty, or mastoidectomy surgery, provided it is discontinued several half-lives (20 minutes or so) before closing or before creation of any enclosed space. The use of a volatile agent and 100% oxygen with intravenous anesthetics is then the acceptable practice until the end of the procedure. Reintroducing nitrous oxide to the inspired gas in the presence of a closed cavity containing air may result in tremendous pressure increases in the middle ear, perhaps greater than 300 mm Hg, and should of course be avoided. The use of nitrous oxide in otolaryngology–head and neck surgery is discussed at length in another article by Irwin and Liang elsewhere in this issue.

Emergence and extubation is another critical part of otolaryngology–head and neck surgery. Head and neck patients often have undergone a hypotensive technique to facilitate delicate middle ear or other otolaryngologic procedures. The use of an LMA for intraoperative management allows a smooth emergence and is discussed in depth by Mandel elsewhere in this issue. However, some patients are not candidates for the LMA and must be intubated for various procedures. In these patients, conventional emergence until awake (with attendant coughing and both arterial and venous hypertension in the head and neck) is to be avoided if possible. At the authors' institution, this is accomplished routinely through selective deep extubation.

The authors consider deep extubation (with spontaneous respiration) if patients (1) are not at increased risk for pulmonary aspiration; (2) have received intravenous metoclopramide and, usually, an antiemetic medication; (3) have had orogastric suction and oropharyngeal suction, and perhaps an intravenous antisialogogue such as glycopyrrolate; (4) have an oropharyngeal airway in place before or immediately after extubation, or (5) have an LMA placed immediately after extubation. The use of an LMA as a bridge to full wakefulness and extubation makes airway management less problematic, especially if the patient has a history or exhibits symptoms of obstructive sleep apnea.

Typically, postoperative patients at the authors' institution are accepted into the post-anesthesia care unit (PACU) with stable respiratory patterns, not yet having entered stage 2 of emergence, with either a Guedel-type oropharyngeal airway or an LMA in place, breathing supplemental oxygen through a low flow apparatus. Caretakers stay with the patient at least one-on-one until the airway has been removed and the patient is awake and responding to commands. Ideally, patients will be awake and oriented and able to show intact nerve VII function, or normal vocalization, shortly after arrival in the PACU.

INTRAOPERATIVE MONITORING OF CRANIAL AND CERVICAL NERVES DURING NECK DISSECTION AND SKULL BASE OPERATIONS

During neck dissection, many nerves and vessels (including the thoracic duct) are at risk.[35–38] Although the usefulness of the NIM tube in monitoring vagus and recurrent laryngeal nerve function is well established, a NIM tube is only helpful in this setting if revision thyroidectomy with neck dissection is undertaken.[37,39] Otherwise, handheld unipolar and bipolar probes are more commonly used to stimulate nerves and observe the movement of target muscles. Typical nerves monitored in neck dissection and skull base surgery are those of the ansa cervicalis or ansa hypoglossi, the phrenic nerve (C3–5), and the lower cranial nerves (VII–XII). **Fig. 4** provides a schematic diagram of the phrenic nerve and ansa cervicalis, and their origins and muscles of innervation. **Table 3** shows the nerves and target innervated muscles that are stimulated and monitored during neck dissection and skull base surgery. Reports of lower cranial nerve pathology[40] or intraoperative monitoring[41] are rare and are mostly anecdotal although Topsakal and colleagues[42] reviewed a series of 123 patients who had IONM of lower cranial nerves during skull base surgery. Details of this report are beyond the scope of this review. Lastly, **Fig. 5** shows a recent application of both IONM and capnography as a means of assessing phrenic (C3–5) function intraoperatively.

The phrenic nerve is at significant risk during cardiac and some otolaryngologic surgeries. Recently,[43] an elegant technique was described for monitoring function of the phrenic nerves through evoked EMG (see **Fig. 5**), in which surgeons stimulated the phrenic nerve using direct visualization during neck surgery for repair of a stretch injury of the brachial plexus. They used a monopolar probe with a constant stimulating current of 2 mA (a typical suprathreshold value used in this setting). The capnograph showed (in the second and third panels of **Fig. 5**) significant evoked diaphragmatic response not palpable or audible through auscultation. However, when the stimulus current reached 7 mA, the diaphragmatic movement ($\gamma = 1$ Hz) was grossly palpable.[43]

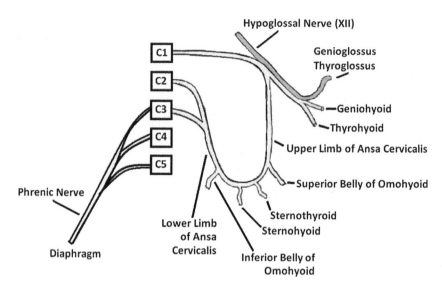

Fig. 4. Schematic of the ansa cervicalis, hypoglossal nerve (XII), and phrenic nerves, and their innervated muscles. These nerves are at risk, and the use of intraoperative nerve monitoring is common, during neck dissections and submandibular region surgeries. The use of a monopolar or bipolar handheld stimulating electrode is common in these kinds of surgeries, and considerations regarding movement, hypotension, positioning, and muscle relaxation are similar to those in other head and neck operations.

Table 3
Cranial nerves and muscles suited for their monitoring in neck dissection and skull base surgery

Cranial Nerve	Muscle
Nerves emerging from the middle cranial fossa	
III	Rectus medialis Rectus inferior
IV	Obliquus superior
V	Digastricus Masseter
VI	Rectus lateralis
Nerves emerging from the posterior cranial fossa	
VII	Frontalis Orbicularis oris Orbicularis oculi Mentalis
IX	Stylopharyngeus
X	Vocalis
XI	Trapezius Sternocleidomastoideus
XII	Hypoglossus Genioglossus

Data from Maurer J, Pelster H, Amedee RG, et al. Intraoperative monitoring of motor cranial nerves in skull base surgery. Skull Base Surg 1995;5:169–75.

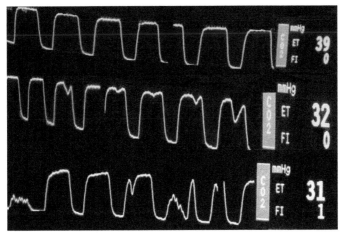

Fig. 5. Fused capnograms as seen on the patient monitor. The top row is a normal capnogram. After phrenic nerve stimulus, the middle row shows notching of the wave form (subclinical diaphragmatic contraction), which degenerates into frank spikes with increasing current corresponding to palpable diaphragmatic contractions. The progressive drop in endtidal carbon dioxide from a baseline of 39 mm Hg to 31 mm Hg is noteworthy. (*Adapted from* Bhagat H, Agarwal A, Sharma MS. Capnography as an aid in localizing the phrenic nerve in brachial plexus Surgery. Technical note. J Brachial Plex Peripher Nerve Inj 2008;3:14; with permission.)

ANESTHETIC CONSIDERATIONS DURING NECK DISSECTION AND SKULL BASE OPERATIONS

Patient movement during neck dissection and skull base surgery may be problematic for several reasons, including its potential to precipitate surgical injury, embolism, or hemorrhage. Assuring adequate depth of anesthesia is important, especially if the Mayfield apparatus or other positioning device is used for craniotomy. Furthermore, if IONM is planned, then muscle relaxants should be used only at induction and intubation. The use of local anesthetics is likewise contraindicated because of their effects on MAP amplitudes and muscle movement. Control of hemostasis during neck dissection is not as critical as during otologic or skull base neurosurgery, but the use of a short-acting opioid infusion such as remifentanil or sufentanil will help control blood pressure and thus help with hemostasis, while also assuring adequate depth of anesthesia. The use of volatile anesthetic agents and nitrous oxide is acceptable only if the nitrous oxide is discontinued well before closing any cavity.

SUMMARY

During otolaryngologic–head and neck surgery, surgeons and anesthesiologists compete for the airway as a part of their cooperative care of the patient. Although it is often brief, this involves intense stimuli (especially to the vocal cords and nearby airway mucosa) alternating with periods of little stimulation. As a goal, anesthetic induction for IONM must be deep enough to ensure patient comfort and lack of awareness, but light enough to allow accurate positioning of a NIM tube, and then immediately deep enough again to prevent coughing and displacement of the tube.

Chirurgie. [Collaborators Identification of the recurrent laryngeal nerve and para-thyroids in thyroid surgery]. Chirurg 2009;80(4):352–63 [in German].

31. Kang SW, Lee S C, Lee SH, et al. Robotic thyroid surgery using a gasless, trans-axillary approach and the da Vinci S system: the operative outcomes of 338 consecutive patients. Surgery 2009;146:1048–55.

32. Dionigi G, Bacuzzi A, Boni L, et al. What is the learning curve for intraoperative neuromonitoring in thyroid surgery? Int J Surg 2008;6(Suppl 1):S7–12.

33. Wheeler AD, Turchiano J, Tobias JD. A case of refractory intraoperative hypoten-sion treated with vasopressin infusion. J Clin Anesth 2008;20:139–42.

34. Witt RL. Facial nerve monitoring in parotid surgery: the standard of care? Otolar-yngol Head Neck Surg 1998;119:468–70.

35. Crile G. Excision of cancer of the head and neck. With special reference to the plan of dissection based on one hundred and thirty-two operations. JAMA 1906;47(22):1780–6.

36. Kurnatowski P, Latkowski B, Lukomski M, et al. Radical neck dissection and the possibility of complications: surgical technique. Otolaryngol Pol 1996;50(4):383–93.

37. Porterfield JR, Factor DA, Grant CS. Operative technique for modified radical neck dissection in papillary thyroid carcinoma. Arch Surg 2009;144(6):567–74.

38. Orhan KS, Demirel T, Baslo B, et al. Spinal accessory nerve function after neck dissections. J Laryngol Otol 2007;121:44–8.

39. Johnson S, Goldenberg D. Intraoperative monitoring of the recurrent laryngeal nerve during revision thyroid surgery. Otolaryngol Clin North Am 2008;41(6): 1147–54.

40. Ceylan S, Karakus A, Durn S, et al. Glossopharyngeal neuralgia: a study of six cases. Neurosurg Rev 1997;20:196–200.

41. Mishler ET, Smith PG. Technical aspects of intraoperative monitoring of lower cranial nerve function. Skull Base Surg 1995;5(4):245–50.

42. Topsakal C, Al-Mefty O, Bulsara KR, et al. Intraoperative monitoring of lower cranial nerves in skull base surgery: technical report and review of 123 monitored cases. Neurosurg Rev 2008;31:45–53.

43. Bhagat H, Agarwal A, Sharma MS. Capnography as an aid in localizing the phrenic nerve in brachial plexus surgery. J Brachial Plex Peripher Nerve Inj 2008;3:14.

Anesthesia, Sleep, and Upper Airway Collapsibility

David R. Hillman, MD[a,b,*], Peter R. Platt, MD[b],
Peter R. Eastwood, PhD[a,c]

KEYWORDS

- Anesthesia • Sleep • Upper airway collapsibility
- Obstructive sleep apnea

Smooth anesthetic induction and emergence is held as an anesthesia management ideal. The term implies a seamless change from the awake to the anesthetized state and back again, based on skillful management of the rate and magnitude of drug administration and attendant issues, including airway management. It conjures up concepts of careful titration to varying concentrations at the site of drug action to produce dose-dependent effects and of the orderly pharmacokinetic processes of absorption, distribution, tissue and receptor binding, and elimination that modulate these changes.

The term does, however, mask the fact that the transition from consciousness to unconsciousness during anesthetic induction is, in neurophysiologic terms at least, quite abrupt,[1] as it is during sleep onset,[2] with a relatively stable state of consciousness or unconsciousness on either side of the transition. Indeed, the thalamocortical pathways involved have been thought to have the characteristics of a bistable flip-flop switch.[2] The transition to unconsciousness is accompanied by an abrupt decrease in upper airway muscle activity and increase in upper airway collapsibility.[3] Hence, on one side of the divide (moderate [conscious] sedation) there is some protection against obstruction afforded by muscle activation and rousability, whereas on the other side (deep [unconscious] sedation) there are vulnerabilities associated with muscle relaxation and, when anesthetized, lack of rousability. Understanding this dichotomy is important in helping plan safe perioperative airway management,

[a] West Australian Sleep Disorders Research Institute, Department of Pulmonary Physiology, Sir Charles Gairdner Hospital, Hospital Avenue, Nedlands, Perth 6009, Western Australia, Australia
[b] Department of Anaesthesia, Sir Charles Gairdner Hospital, Hospital Avenue, Nedlands, Perth, Western Australia, Australia
[c] School of Anatomy and Human Biology, University of Western Australia, Stirling Highway, Perth, Western Australia, Australia
* Corresponding author. West Australian Sleep Disorders Research Institute, Department of Pulmonary Physiology, Sir Charles Gairdner Hospital, Hospital Avenue, Nedlands, Perth 6009, Western Australia, Australia.
E-mail address: David.Hillman@health.wa.gov.au

Anesthesiology Clin 28 (2010) 443–455
doi:10.1016/j.anclin.2010.07.003
1932-2275/10/$ – see front matter © 2010 Elsevier Inc. All rights reserved.

especially where there is particular vulnerability to obstruction, as with obstructive sleep apnea (OSA).

REGULATION OF CONSCIOUSNESS

An ascending arousal system originating in the brainstem is crucial in maintaining wakefulness with well-defined cell groups involved in 2 major pathways.[2] The major inputs into one of these are the upper pontine pedunculopontine and laterodorsal tegmental nuclei. These activate thalamic relay neurons and the thalamic reticular nucleus that are crucial for transmission of information to the cerebral cortex. The other pathway originates in centers in the upper brainstem and caudal hypothalamus, including the locus coeruleus, dorsal and median raphe nuclei, ventral periaqueductal gray matter, and the tuberomammillary nucleus. This ascending arousal pathway bypasses the thalamus, activating pathways in the lateral hypothalamus and basal forebrain and then the cerebral cortex.

The activity of these wakefulness-promoting pathways is inhibited by a system of gamma-aminobutyric acid (GABA)-containing neurons, in which the lateral hypothalamic ventrolateral preoptic nucleus (VLPO) appears to play a key role. It both receives afferents from and has outputs to the major cell groups in the brainstem and hypothalamus that participate in arousal. These pathways have mutually inhibitory influences on each other (**Fig. 1**).[4] During wakefulness the activity of the VLPO is strongly inhibited by the locus coeruleus and other wakefulness-promoting centers. As the activity of these decreases at sleep onset, the VLPO becomes active, in turn reciprocally inhibiting their activity. These mutually inhibitory elements set up a self-reinforcing loop whereby activity on one side inhibits activity on the other, acting to disinhibit its own activity. This activity has the characteristic of a bistable flip-flop switch that acts to produce stable states of wakefulness or sleep with sharp transitions between them.[2] Relevant to anesthesia, the VLPO is heavily populated by GABA type A-ergic neurons and anesthetic agents (eg, propofol) potentiate its GABAergic inhibition of

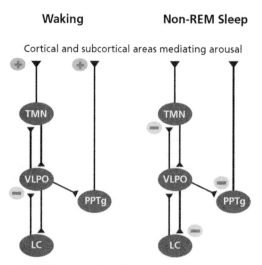

Fig. 1. Some connections of the ventrolateral preoptic nucleus involved in the regulation of sleep and wakefulness. TMN, tuberomammillary nucleus; LC, locus coeruleus; PPTg, pedunculopontine tegmental nuclei. (*From* Harrison NL. General anesthesia research: aroused from a deep sleep? Nature Neuroscience 2002;5:928; with permission.)

arousal pathways through stimulatory effects on $GABA_A$ receptors, and perhaps by facilitating excitatory inputs into the VLPO.[5] Hence, the sleep switch is also activated by anesthetic agents and may constitute a narcotic mechanism that is common to sleep and anesthesia.[1,4]

Consistent with this threshold-related switching behavior wake-sleep and sleep-wake transitions are abrupt as are transitions from consciousness to unconsciousness during induction of anesthesia.[1,3] An essential difference between the sleep and anesthetized states is, of course, that with sleep following the flip to unconsciousness, moderate stimulation is then sufficient to disturb sleep causing a flop to consciousness; whereas once anesthetic drug-induced unconsciousness is induced, the capacity to arouse requires at least some drug elimination to occur before it is restored.

Consciousness provides protection for upper airway patency and respiration. The wakeful state provides a nonspecific behavioral drive to respiration and to the upper airway musculature, enhancing tonic and phasic neuronal activation. It is the loss of this activation with sleep or anesthesia-induced unconsciousness that is responsible for increased collapsibility of the upper airway[3] and the obstruction that ensues in predisposed, unprotected individuals. In sleep obstruction of the upper airway is terminated by arousal, accompanied by muscle activation and restoration of patency with repetitive events forming the basis of OSA. In anesthesia, such obstructive events require active intervention by attending staff at least until the ability to arouse spontaneously is restored.

DETERMINANTS OF UPPER AIRWAY PATENCY

Upper airway obstruction during sleep or anesthesia results from a combination of an anatomically predisposed airway and the permissive effect of the muscle relaxation that is an inevitable consequence of these states. Anatomic predisposition can be thought of in terms of caliber and shape of the airway, extraluminal tissue pressure, and airway wall compliance. Obstruction is most likely to occur where substantial anatomic predisposition is present, posture is unfavorable (supine, mouth open, neck flexed), and muscle relaxation is profound (as in anesthesia or rapid eye movement [REM] sleep). The tendency to collapse is countered by upper airway muscle activation.

Caliber of the Airway

There are several reasons why a narrow airway is more vulnerable to collapse. First, and most obviously, the smaller the airway the less is the absolute change in luminal cross section required for airway closure. Second, Laplace's law dictates that at equilibrium the transmural pressure across a concave surface is directly proportional to wall tension and inversely proportional to its radius of curvature. It follows that the transmural pressure gradient required to prevent collapse of the airway varies inversely with its radius of curvature. Third, increased resistance of the narrowed airway necessitates generation of more negative intraluminal pressures. Fourth, airway wall compliance is increased at lower calibers (**Fig. 2**).[6]

Transluminal Pressure Gradient

The pressure gradient across the pharyngeal wall is determined by the difference between the pressure in the tissues surrounding the airway (the extraluminal tissue pressure) and the pressure within the airway lumen (intraluminal pressure). The extraluminal tissue pressure increases with obesity and other increases in tissue volume, such as edema, or with narrowing of skeletal confines, as with neck flexion or micrognathia or retrognathia.[7] Intraluminal pressure decreases during inspiration and

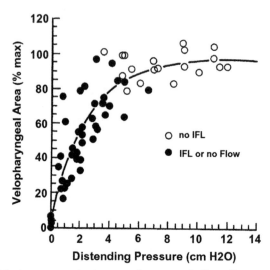

Fig. 2. Relationship between velopharyngeal area and distending pressure in humans. Compliance (slope of the relationship) increases at low calibers. IFL, inspiratory flow limitation. (*Adapted from* Isono S, Morrison DL, Launois SH, et al. Static mechanics of the velopharynx of patients with obstructive sleep apnea. J Appl Physiol 1993;75:148–54; with permission.)

increases during expiration. The magnitude of the inspiratory decrease is a function of inspiratory flow rate and of resistance upstream of the site of interest. It becomes greater, for example, with increased nasal resistance.

Compliance of the Airway Wall

Pharyngeal wall compliance is a measure of its degree of flaccidity and, in the absence of muscle activity, reflects its intrinsic elastic properties and the degree of radial (transverse) and axial (longitudinal) tension to which it is subjected. A more compliant (flaccid) airway is more likely to collapse and, indeed, compliance is increased in OSA.[6] The properties of connective tissue, bone, and fat all influence intrinsic compliance, as does surface tension.[8] Compliance tends to increase at low calibers, increasing collapsibility (see **Fig. 2**).[6] Longitudinal tension on the airway increases with increasing lung volume (tracheal tug), acting to decrease compliance.[9] This activity, along with reflex muscle activation (see later discussion), stabilizes the airway during inspiration.

Upper Airway Muscle Activation

Inspiratory activation of pharyngeal dilator muscles, of which the genioglossus is the most important and best studied, counteracts the narrowing effect of the inspiration-associated decreases in intraluminal pressure. In addition to this phasic inspiratory activity, tonic activity is present during wakefulness to help stiffen and stabilize the airway wall. The activity of the genioglossus (and other extrinsic tongue muscles, apart from palatoglossus) is mediated via the hypoglossal nerve. Its nucleus is situated in the medulla and receives a variety of inputs that together determine its output.[10] These inputs include negative pressure reflexes initiated by mechanoreceptors principally situated in the larynx, phasic inspiratory input from respiratory neurons arising from the pontomedullary central pattern generator, and a tonic excitatory stimulus related to the wakeful state. Each of these inputs is depressed by sleep or anesthesia to a varying degree through central effects, with muscle relaxants providing an additional peripheral component in cases where they are used. Hence, accounting for all of the inputs is important when considering the effects of sleep and anesthesia on upper airway behavior.

THE NATURE OF OBSTRUCTIVE SLEEP APNEA

With sleep, upper airway collapsibility increases as a result of a reduction in pharyngeal dilator muscle activation and loss of lung volume, which decreases longitudinal traction on it. The reduction in muscle activation appears to be the combined result of loss of the stimulatory effect of wakefulness, reduction in respiratory drive, and depression of negative pressure reflexes. These changes are evident at sleep onset but vary in intensity with sleep state, being more profound in REM than non-REM sleep. Although the accompanying increase in upper airway collapsibility with sleep is present in everyone, in normal individuals without anatomic compromise, the upper airway is robust and patency is not significantly compromised. However, in individuals with anatomically vulnerable airways, these changes can precipitate partial or complete upper airway obstruction. Indeed patients with OSA appear to have a relative increase in wakeful upper airway muscle activation to compensate for their anatomic predisposition to obstruction.[11]

OSA is characterized by recurrent episodes of partial or complete upper airway obstruction during sleep. These obstructive hypopneas and apneas are associated with hypoxemia and sympathetic activation and are terminated by arousals, which disrupt sleep and are responsible for the excessive daytime sleepiness that usually accompanies it. Loud habitual snoring is a usual, but not invariable, associated feature that signifies the presence of a narrow, floppy airway. Hypoxia may also accompany the respiratory disturbances; its magnitude varies with the length of the disturbance, lung volume (and therefore size of oxygen stores), and degree of intrapulmonary shunt. Although magnitude of hypoxemia and extent of symptoms are important, severity of OSA is usually expressed in terms of the number of apneas and hypopneas per hour of sleep, the apnea-hypopnea index. In adults, less than 5 respiratory events per hour of sleep is considered normal, 5 to 15 mild, 15 to 30 moderate, and greater than 30 severe OSA.[12] Sleep is not a homogenous state and severity of OSA varies with sleep stage, body posture, and neck position. It is worse in REM than non-REM sleep and is aggravated in the supine posture or when the neck is flexed. In milder cases, the problem may only be apparent when the individual is in supine REM sleep.

A total of 4% of adults have OSA to a clinically significant degree.[13] Everyday consequences of the problem include the social costs of the loud snoring that often accompanies it; the excessive daytime sleepiness that results from recurrent arousals with its negative implications for safety, productivity and social interactions; and various comorbidities, including hypertension and vascular disease, diabetes and metabolic syndrome, and mood disorders. Addressing predisposing lifestyle issues, such as obesity and sedative or alcohol abuse, are important. Beyond addressing these issues, as long as no medically or surgically correctible predisposing abnormality exists, the treatment of choice is continuous positive airway pressure therapy delivered by a nasal or face mask.[14] Dental splints designed to hold the mandible forward during sleep are a useful but less predictably effective alternative.[15]

The primary site of collapse within the upper airway during sleep is the velopharynx in the majority of patients (approximately 80%), as it is during anesthesia.[16,17] The other common site of collapse is retrolingual. These vulnerable segments correspond to the narrowest levels within the upper airway.[18]

Factors that act to narrow the airway predispose to OSA. These factors include increasing age,[19] male gender[20] (with male [central] distribution of body fat important), menopause,[21] obesity,[22] increased neck circumference,[23] macroglossia,[24] retrognathia,[25] and maxillary constriction.[26] These factors may be present to varying degrees in otherwise normal individuals or they may be part of a disease syndrome, such as acromegaly, Down's syndrome, Pierre-Robin syndrome, or other syndromes associated with craniofacial abnormality. There is an association with difficult intubation and indeed many of the features that suggest a difficult airway from the anesthesia point of view, either difficult intubation or difficult mask ventilation, also suggest OSA.[27,28]

Obesity exerts its effects through increasing local compressive forces on the upper airway and by decreasing functional residual capacity, and therefore longitudinal traction on the upper airway, particularly when recumbent.[22] There are familial predispositions to OSA.[29] Neuromuscular conditions affecting the upper airway muscles also predispose to OSA[30] as do endocrine (hypothyroidism, acromegaly), connective tissue, and storage diseases that decrease upper airway caliber. Specific pathologies in the upper airway also predispose to obstruction at discrete sites. These pathologies include nasal obstruction,[31] tonsillar and adenoidal hypertrophy,[32] pharyngeal tumors, foreign bodies, hematomas, and edema. Stroke and head injury can increase vulnerability to OSA by depressing muscle tone and arousal responses, as can alcohol[33] and sedative consumption.[34] Various sleep postures increase vulnerability to obstruction, including supine recumbency,[35] neck flexion,[36] and mouth opening.

OSA AND PERIOPERATIVE RISK

The factors that predispose to OSA also predispose to obstruction under anesthesia and those with OSA are prone to difficulties with tracheal intubation and with airway maintenance under anesthesia.[27] There is a relative paucity of studies of perioperative risk relating to OSA and so published guidelines, such as the American Society of Anesthesiologists guidelines,[37] remain heavily dependent on expert opinion rather than high-level evidence. Nevertheless, the available literature does suggest some trends that appear consistent with pathophysiological considerations.

A large retrospective case control study found that OSA did not appear to be a risk factor for unanticipated admissions in outpatient surgery; there was no difference in perioperative adverse events or unplanned admissions between subjects with OSA and matched controls.[38] When the reasons for such unplanned admissions were analyzed there was no clear difference in profiles of causes between the groups. However, when major surgery is considered a different picture emerges; a retrospective case control study of postoperative morbidity after hip or knee arthroplasty demonstrated a substantial increase in complications, particularly serious complications, including those requiring unplanned intensive care unit admission, in subjects with OSA.[39] It showed an increased length of hospital stay for these subjects. These findings are supported by another retrospective matched cohort study that suggests that the risk of postoperative complications for patients with diagnosed OSA is double that of patients without this diagnosis.[40] Risks associated with upper airway surgery appear to increase in the presence of OSA; in adults post-uvulopalatopharyngoplasty respiratory complications appear to be associated with more severe OSA.[41] A study of children undergoing adenotonsillectomy for OSA versus those undergoing this procedure for other reasons demonstrated an increase in complications in the immediate perioperative period for the OSA subgroup, including problems during induction of anesthesia, emergence from it, and in early recovery.[42] Although a far greater body of literature is required, these findings suggest that, at least for minor procedures, the major risks relating to OSA status are likely to be found in the immediate perioperative period, with patients undergoing upper airway surgery at particular risk. This finding may particularly be the case with children given their narrow upper airways and low functional residual capacities, which act to limit oxygen stores relative to metabolic requirement when in the obstructed state. It may be that the risks relating to major surgery relate to the requirement for postoperative sedative and narcotic analgesics in many of these patients, with an attendant risk of impaired consciousness (either through direct drug effect or through respiratory depression and hypercapnia) and depressed arousal responses. These observations are consistent with the notion that the perioperative and postoperative problems for patients with OSA particularly relate to unconsciousness and suppression of arousal responses and that their risk profile diminishes substantially with return of consciousness and rousability following anesthesia, providing they are not further compromised by subsequent drug administration.

The return of ready rousability is an important criterion to be met before discharge from the recovery room following anesthesia for patients without other cause for prolonged unconsciousness. Although emergence from anesthesia can be accompanied by abrupt return of consciousness[43] (again suggesting the threshold switchlike behavior at the interface between consciousness and unconsciousness), often this is not the case, which reflects persistent sedative drug activity in some cases. However, it is also probable that anesthesia frequently transposes into natural sleep when postoperative pain in not an issue, particularly late at night when propensity to natural sleep is the greatest. This factor may not be readily recognized given the similarities in behavioral appearances between sleep and anesthesia.

In outpatient surgery, discharge from the recovery room is followed by discharge home, within a few hours, once the effects of the anesthetic drugs have dissipated. However, with more invasive surgery, the substantial postoperative analgesia/sedation that is often required means that vulnerable patients remains at risk of upper airway obstruction through its depressant effects on rousability. Regional anesthetic techniques allow some of this potential difficulty to be circumvented. Although anesthesia itself appears to have some restorative properties when unmodified by the effects of surgery,[44] sleep is usually disturbed in the postoperative period. The degree of this disturbance varies with type and extent of surgery, pain and its treatment, personality, and the nursing environment. It is characterized by sleep restriction or deprivation, sleep fragmentation, and distorted sleep architecture with loss of REM sleep and may persist for many days postoperatively.[45] These disturbances can result in cognitive and psychomotor dysfunction.[46] These disturbances cause 2 problems for patients with OSA: (1) the effects of the postoperative sleep fragmentation compound those of fragmentation caused by OSA itself, and (2) re-establishment of normal sleep after a substantial period of sleep deprivation is characterized by a state of "REM-sleep rebound" during which the proportion of REM sleep increases above the usual adult proportion of 20% to 25% of total sleep time.[45] This state may last 1 or more nights. Given that REM sleep is the most vulnerable stage of sleep for depression of neural drive to the upper airway, the overall severity of OSA can be aggravated by it.

OSA AND ANESTHESIA MANAGEMENT

Anesthesia management of patients with OSA must ensure that their particular vulnerability when unconscious or under the influence of sedative drugs is adequately addressed (**Box 1**). The potential vulnerability of patients with OSA is a matter of concern to anesthesiologists and has led to the development of guidelines for the

---

Box 1
OSA and anesthesia management

- Try to identify OSA preoperatively.

- When not previously diagnosed, refer patients for preoperative evaluation of sleep where the probability of OSA is high, surgery is elective, and there is a likely need for postoperative narcotic analgesia or sedation.

- When previously diagnosed and compliant with CPAP, ensure it is available for perioperative use.

- Where previously diagnosed but not compliant with CPAP, reinstruct in its use.

- Avoid sedative premedication.

- Use regional anesthesia and analgesia where feasible.

- When general anesthesia is used, be prepared for difficult intubation and other difficulties in airway maintenance. Use techniques that allow early return of consciousness.

- Try to minimize postoperative sedation.

- Have CPAP available for early postoperative use.

- Nurse in a high-dependency area with continuous monitoring until patients are sentient and able to self-administer CPAP. Patients requiring ongoing narcotic analgesia or sedation should remain in a high-dependency area until this need abates.

- Use lateral positioning, a nasopharyngeal airway, and oxygen therapy where CPAP is refused and upper airway obstruction is problematic.

- Consider OSA in patients with difficult airways perioperatively. Inform patients and refer for investigation for the possibility where clinically indicated.

---

perioperative management of OSA by organizations, such as the American Society of Anesthesiologists.[37] Principles addressed in such guidelines include systematic identification of patients at risk; avoidance of sedation in unsupervised surroundings; minimization of use of sedative and narcotic drugs; preparation for difficulties in intubation and airway management intraoperatively and immediately postoperatively; careful postoperative supervision until sentient; use of postoperative aids, such artificial airways or continuous positive airway pressure (CPAP) therapy where airway compromise exists; and particular care following upper airway surgery.

Identifying OSA Preoperatively

Patients with OSA may present with the diagnosis made and, better still, treatment instituted. However, at least as commonly given the notorious underdiagnosis of the problem, individuals with OSA present undiagnosed. A fairly simple collection of symptoms and signs will alert the vigilant anesthesiologist to the possibility of the disorder during preoperative evaluation. The cardinal symptoms of OSA are habitual snoring, witnessed apnea, disrupted and unrefreshing sleep, and excessive daytime sleepiness. Not all of these features are present in all patients, but any combination of them in an individual is highly suggestive of the presence of this common and potentially disabling disorder. Signs include obesity, increased neck circumference, mandibular or maxillary hypoplasia, oropharyngeal crowding (high Mallampati scores, decreased pharyngeal width), and hypertension. Any signs that suggest to an anesthesiologist that there may be difficulties with tracheal intubation or with airway maintenance perioperatively should also suggest OSA. The converse also holds; symptoms and signs of OSA should alert the anesthesiologist to the possibility of difficulties with airway management. Clearly these symptoms and signs should be sought at preoperative evaluation, as should the history of prior diagnosis of the problem. Indeed, apart from the importance of observations made during preoperative evaluation and intraoperatively for perioperative management, they can also help identify previously undiagnosed OSA, with long-term benefits for patients. The relationship between OSA and airway collapsibility under deep sedation is utilized in sleep nasendoscopy. This procedure is performed under drug-induced sedation to assess upper airway collapsibility and identify the likely primary site of obstruction for subsequent surgical attention.[47]

When Possible OSA has not been Previously Diagnosed

When the possibility of previously undiagnosed OSA has been raised by preoperative evaluation, the probability of its presence can be assessed using a prediction rule approach, such as that of Flemons.[48] Surgery should be postponed when this assessment indicates an intermediate or high likelihood of OSA or the anesthesiologist is otherwise concerned and surgery is elective and likely to require narcotic analgesia or sedation postoperatively. When postponed, patients should be referred to a sleep physician for evaluation and, where indicated, initiation of appropriate treatment.

When OSA has been Previously Diagnosed and Patients are Compliant with CPAP Therapy

Patients with diagnosed OSA on CPAP therapy should be instructed to bring their equipment to the hospital for use whenever asleep or sedated.

When OSA has been Previously Diagnosed and Patients are not Compliant with CPAP Therapy

Patients who have been diagnosed with OSA, either independently or as part of preoperative workup, but who do not use CPAP regularly, should be reinstructed in its use preoperatively, so that it is readily applicable whenever under the influence of narcotics or sedatives.

Avoidance of Sedative Premedication

Premedication with sedatives or opioids should be avoided wherever possible when OSA is known or suspected. When these substances are required because of anxiety or pain, patients should be observed in a high-dependency area.

Anesthetic Technique

Regional anesthetic and analgesic techniques should be used where feasible. When general anesthesia is needed, the possibility of difficult intubation and difficulties with airway management must be considered. Technique and drugs used should be selected to allow early return of consciousness and minimal postanesthetic sedation whenever possible. CPAP must be available for immediate use postoperatively in all patients with known or suspected OSA. Indeed, CPAP or noninvasive bilevel ventilation should be considered for use during procedures involving moderate/deep sedation to maintain airway patency, particularly when patients are familiar with these therapies.

Postoperative Nursing Environment

Patients diagnosed with OSA, or when the suspicion of it has arisen preoperatively (but not been investigated because of emergency), intraoperatively (because of difficulty with tracheal intubation or maintenance of airway patency), or in the recovery room, must be nursed in a high-dependency area postoperatively with appropriate monitoring, including continuous oximetry. This monitoring should continue until patients are sentient and able to reliably administer CPAP unassisted or, in cases where OSA has only been suspected, airway stability during sleep or sedation has been confirmed. Patients with ongoing requirement for postoperative narcotic analgesia or sedation should remain in a high-dependency nursing environment until this need abates. Particular care is required after upper airway surgery because postoperative edema may temporarily worsen upper airway patency, even after operations aimed at increasing pharyngeal caliber, such as laser-assisted uvulopalatoplasty.[49]

When CPAP therapy is refused and upper airway obstruction continues to be problematic, use of lateral positioning, a nasopharyngeal airway, and oxygen therapy are alternate but less satisfactory strategies. In some settings, such as when the nose is packed postoperatively, a face mask rather than a nasal mask will need to be used to deliver CPAP. In other settings, such as surgery involving the sino-nasal tract and skull base (eg, pituitary surgery), early use of CPAP postoperatively may be undesirable because of concerns regarding a potential for pneumocephalus.

Postdischarge Management

When suspicion of previously undiagnosed OSA has arisen as a result of preoperative, intraoperative, or postoperative events, patients should be informed and referred to a sleep physician for further investigation.

SUMMARY

Patients with OSA have airways that are difficult when unconscious, whether the unconsciousness is a result of sleep or anesthesia. Anesthesia presents particular problems for such patients because, unlike during sleep, protection afforded by the ability to arouse is suppressed. Furthermore, anesthesia is associated with profound muscle relaxation, whereas during sleep some muscle activation is retained during non-REM sleep. These particular vulnerabilities are present until consciousness returns and must be accounted for in perioperative anesthesia management. OSA is underdiagnosed and its prevalence continues to increase in advanced economies as obesity and age increases. Careful preoperative evaluation and insightful perioperative observation is likely to identify patients at risk, highlighting the need for both careful postoperative management and specific follow-up to ensure that the sleep-related component of the difficult airway receives appropriate care.

REFERENCES

1. Franks NP. General anaesthesia: from molecular targets to neuronal pathways of sleep and arousal. Nat Rev Neurosci 2008;9:370–86.
2. Saper CB, Scammell TE, Lu J. Hypothalamic regulation of sleep and circadian rhythms. Nature 2005;437:1257–63.
3. Hillman DR, Walsh JH, Maddison KJ, et al. Evolution of changes in upper airway collapsibility during slow induction of anesthesia with propofol. Anesthesiology 2009;111:63–71.
4. Harrison NL. General anesthesia research: aroused from a deep sleep? Nat Neurosci 2002;5:928–9.
5. Li KY, Guan Y, Krnjevic K, et al. Propofol facilitates glutamatergic transmission to the neurons of the ventrolateral preoptic nucleus. Anesthesiology 2009;111: 1271–8.

6. Isono S, Morrison DL, Launois SH, et al. Static mechanics of the velopharynx of patients with obstructive sleep apnea. J Appl Physiol 1993;75:148–54.

7. Watanabe T, Isono S, Tanaka A, et al. Contribution of body habitus and craniofacial characteristics to segmental closing pressures of the passive pharynx in patients with sleep-disordered breathing. Am J Respir Crit Care Med 2002;165: 260–5.

8. Kirkness J, Madronio M, Stavrinou R, et al. Relationship between surface tension of upper airway lining liquid and upper airway collapsibility during sleep in obstructive sleep apnea hypopnea syndrome. J Appl Physiol 2003;95:1761–6.

9. Stanchina M, Malhotra A, Fogel RB, et al. The influence of lung volume on pharyngeal mechanics, collapsibility, and genioglossus muscle activation during sleep. Sleep 2003;26:851–6.

10. White DP. Pathogenesis of obstructive and central sleep apnea. Am J Respir Crit Care Med 2005;172:1363–70.

11. Mezzanotte WS, Tangel DJ, White DP. Waking genioglossal electromyogram in sleep apnea patients versus normal controls (a neuromuscular compensatory mechanism). J Clin Invest 1992;89:1571–9.

12. Practice parameters for the indications for polysomnography and related procedures. Polysomnography Task Force, American Sleep Disorders Association Standards of Practice Committee. Sleep 1997;20:406–22.

13. Young T, Palta M, Dempsey J, et al. The occurrence of sleep-disordered breathing among middle-aged adults. N Engl J Med 1993;328:1230–5.

14. Sullivan CE, Issa FG, Berthon-Jones M, et al. Reversal of obstructive sleep apnoea by continuous positive airway pressure applied through the nares. Lancet 1981;18:862–5.

15. O'Sullivan RA, Hillman DR, Mateljan R, et al. Mandibular advancement splint: an appliance to treat snoring and obstructive sleep apnea. Am J Respir Crit Care Med 1995;151:194–8.

16. Morrison DL, Launois SH, Isono S, et al. Pharyngeal narrowing and closing pressures in patients with obstructive sleep apnea. Am Rev Respir Dis 1993;148: 606–11.

17. Eastwood PR, Szollosi I, Platt PR, et al. Collapsibility of the upper airway during anesthesia with isoflurane. Anesthesiology 2002;97:786–93.

18. Isono S, Remmers JE, Tanaka A, et al. Anatomy of pharynx in patients with obstructive sleep apnea and in normal subjects. J Appl Physiol 1997;82:1319–26.

19. Malhotra A, Huang Y, Fogel R, et al. Aging influences on pharyngeal anatomy and physiology: the predisposition to pharyngeal collapse. Am J Med 2006;119: e9–14.

20. Malhotra A, Huang Y, Fogel RB, et al. The male predisposition to pharyngeal collapse: importance of airway length. Am J Respir Crit Care Med 2002;166: 1388–95.

21. Dancey DR, Haly PJ, Soong C, et al. Impact of menopause on the prevalence and severity of sleep apnea. Chest 2001;120:151–5.

22. Young T, Peppard PE, Taheri S. Excess weight and sleep disordered breathing. J Appl Physiol 2005;99:1592–9.

23. Davies RJ, Stradling JR. The relationship between neck circumference, radiographic pharyngeal anatomy, and the obstructive sleep apnoea syndrome. Eur Respir J 1990;3:509–14.

24. Schellenberg JB, Maislin G, Schwab RJ. Physical findings and the risk for obstructive sleep apnea. The importance of oropharyngeal structures. Am J Respir Crit Care Med 2000;162:740–8.

25. Tangugsorn V, Skatvedt O, Krogstad O, et al. Obstructive sleep apnoea: a cephalometric study. Part I. Cervico-craniofacial skeletal morphology. Eur J Orthod 1995;17:45–56.
26. Cistulli P, Richards GN, Palmisano RG, et al. Influence of maxillary constriction on nasal resistance and sleep apnea severity in patients with Marfan's syndrome. Chest 1996;110:1184–8.
27. Hiremath AS, Hillman DR, James AL, et al. Relationship between difficult tracheal intubation and obstructive sleep apnoea. Br J Anaesth 1998;80:606–11.
28. Kheterpal S, Han R, Tremper KK, et al. Incidence and predictors of difficult and impossible mask ventilation. Anesthesiology 2006;105:885–91.
29. Redline S, Tosteson T, Tishler PV, et al. Studies in the genetics of obstructive sleep apnoea. Familial aggregation of symptoms associated with sleep related breathing disturbances. Am Rev Respir Dis 1992;145:440–4.
30. Guilleminault C, Stoohs R, Quera-Salva MA. Sleep-related obstructive and non-obstructive apneas and neurologic disorders. Neurology 1992;42:53–60.
31. Rappai M, Collop N, Kemp S, et al. The nose and sleep-disordered breathing: what we know and what we do not know. Chest 2003;124:2309–23.
32. Helfaer MA, Wilson MD. Obstructive sleep apnea, control of ventilation, and anesthesia in children. Pediatr Clin North Am 1994;41:131–51.
33. Taasan VC, Block AJ, Boysen PG, et al. Alcohol increases sleep apnea and oxygen desaturation in asymptomatic men. Am J Med 1981;71:240–5.
34. Berry RB, Kouchi K, Bower J, et al. Triazolam in patients with obstructive sleep apnea. Am J Respir Crit Care Med 1995;151:450–4.
35. Penzel T, Moller M, Becker HF, et al. Effect of sleep position and sleep stage on the collapsibility of the upper airways in patients with sleep apnea. Sleep 2001; 24:90–5.
36. Walsh JH, Maddison KJ, Platt PR, et al. Influence of head extension, flexion, and rotation on collapsibility of the passive upper airway. Sleep 2008;31:1440–7.
37. Gross JB, Bachenberg KL, Benumof JL. American Society of Anesthesiologists Task Force on Perioperative management of patients with obstructive sleep apnea: practice guidelines for the perioperative management of patients with obstructive sleep apnea. Anesthesiology 2006;104:1081–91.
38. Sabers C, Plevak DJ, Schroeder DR, et al. The diagnosis of obstructive sleep apnea as a risk factor for unanticipated admissions in outpatient surgery. Anesth Analg 2003;96:1328–35.
39. Gupta RM, Parvizi J, Hanssen AD, et al. Postoperative complications in patients with obstructive sleep apnea syndrome undergoing hip or knee replacement: a case-control study. Mayo Clin Proc 2001;76:897–905.
40. Liao P, Yegneswaran B, Vairavanathan S, et al. Postoperative complications in patients with obstructive sleep apnea: a retrospective matched cohort study. Can J Anaesth 2009;56:819–28.
41. Kim JA, Lee JJ, Jung HH. Predictive factors of immediate postoperative complications after uvulopalatopharyngoplasty. Laryngoscope 2005;115:1837–40.
42. Sanders JC, King MA, Mitchell RB, et al. Perioperative complications of adenotonsillectomy in children with obstructive sleep apnea syndrome. Anesth Analg 2006;103:1115–21.
43. Doi M, Gajraj RJ, Mantzaridis H, et al. Relationship between calculated blood concentration of propofol and electrophysiological variables during emergence from anaesthesia: comparison of bispectral index, spectral edge frequency, median frequency and auditory evoked potential index. Br J Anaesth 1997;78: 180–4.

44. Tung A, Mendelson WB. Anesthesia and sleep. Sleep Med Rev 2004;8:213–25.
45. Knill RL, Moote CA, Skinner MI, et al. Anesthesia with abdominal surgery leads to intense REM sleep during the first postoperative week. Anesthesiology 1990;70: 52–61.
46. Treggiari-Venzi M, Borgeat A, Fuchs-Buder T, et al. Overnight sedation with midazolam or propofol in the ICU: effects on sleep quality, anxiety and depression. Intensive Care Med 1996;22:1186–90.
47. Rodriguez-Bruno K, Goldberg AN, McCulloch CE, et al. Test-retest reliability of drug-induced sleep endoscopy. Otolaryngol Head Neck Surg 2009;140:646–51.
48. Flemons WW. Obstructive sleep apnea. N Engl J Med 2002;347:498–504.
49. Terris DJ, Clerk AA, Norbash AM, et al. Characterization of post-operative edema following laser assisted uvulopalatoplasty using MRI and polysomnography. Laryngoscope 2009;106:124–8.

Regional Anesthesia for Office-based Procedures in Otorhinolaryngology

Deya N. Jourdy, MD, Ashutosh Kacker, MD*

KEYWORDS

- Local anesthesia • Regional anesthesia • Topical anesthesia
- Otolaryngology • Otorhinolaryngology • Head and neck

Local and topical anesthetic techniques have long been used for office-based procedures in the specialty of otorhinolaryngology. In fact, before the advent of safer intravenous and inhaled general anesthetic techniques, many procedures now mainly performed under general anesthesia (ie, rhinoplasty, rhytidectomy, and tonsillectomy) were performed with the use of local and topical anesthesia. Tonsillectomy, presently one of the most commonly performed surgical procedures in the United States, is still performed under local anesthesia by some otorhinolaryngologists.[1,2] There are numerous advantages to using local and topical anesthesia for office-based procedures, including a shorter recovery period and the maintenance of a conscious patient who can communicate with the surgeon and maintain his or her own airway during the procedure. Furthermore, in the current age of rising health care costs, the use of local and topical anesthetic techniques for office-based procedures can be an effective means to deliver less expensive, high-quality medical care. Paramount to the success of these procedures is patient selection. The patient must be cooperative, willing to follow precise instructions, and willing to remain awake for the procedure. With this in mind, numerous procedures can be performed on the external face, ear, nose, oral cavity, nasopharynx, oropharynx, hypopharynx, and larynx, using either local or topical anesthetic techniques, or a combination of both.

Infiltration of local anesthetic, such as lidocaine, into structures of the head and neck can be extremely painful for the patient because of the abundance of highly sensitive tissues. To reduce the discomfort often associated with the local blocks that are reviewed later in this article, the physician should consider buffering acidic anesthetic agents with 7.5% sodium bicarbonate solution in a 1:5 dilution by volume (eg, 1 mL 7.5% sodium bicarbonate and 5 mL 1% lidocaine).[3] Infiltration should be

Department of Otorhinolaryngology, Weill Cornell Medical College, 1305 York Avenue, 5th Floor, New York, NY 10021, USA
* Corresponding author.
E-mail address: ask9001@med.cornell.edu

Anesthesiology Clin 28 (2010) 457–468
doi:10.1016/j.anclin.2010.07.004
1932-2275/10/$ – see front matter © 2010 Elsevier Inc. All rights reserved.

performed in a slow and steady manner using a fine needle such as a 27-gauge needle or smaller and placed within the dermal-subdermal or mucosal-submucosal plane to lessen pain from soft tissue dissection by the local anesthetic.[4]

EAR
External Ear

Indications for local anesthesia of the auricle include repair of a torn lobule, examination and treatment of traumatic lacerations, and treatment of auricular hematomas. When anesthetizing the external ear with regional blocks, the addition of epinephrine to the anesthetic solution should be used with caution if there is severe devascularization of the tissue, as this may result in tissue necrosis. However, the use of epinephrine may be of great benefit, as it reduces bleeding and prolongs anesthesia, and there is no good evidence that shows harm in its use. In fact, one study looking at more than 10,000 patients undergoing nasal and ear surgery showed that the addition of epinephrine to the anesthetic solution had a relatively small influence on blood perfusion and resulted in no cases of tissue necrosis.[5]

Several techniques can be used to accomplish anesthesia of the auricle. To achieve anesthesia of the posteromedial, posterolateral, and inferior auricle, local anesthetic, such as 1% lidocaine, can be injected in the posterior sulcus of the auricle (**Fig. 1**). Injection in this location will block branches of the greater auricular nerve and lesser occipital nerve that supply sensory innervation to the auricle. If anesthesia of the anterosuperior and anteromedial portions of the auricle is desired, a block of the auriculotemporal nerve can be performed by injecting local anesthetic just superior and anterior to the tragus. Alternatively, local anesthetic can be injected in a diamond formation around the auricle to achieve a field block of the external ear (**Fig. 2**).[6]

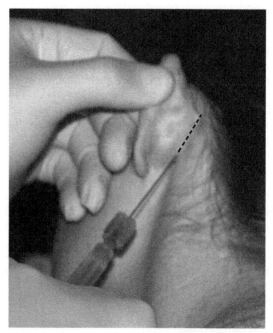

Fig. 1. Injection of local anesthetic in the crescent-shaped retroauricular sulcus provides anesthesia of the posteromedial, posterolateral, and inferior auricle.

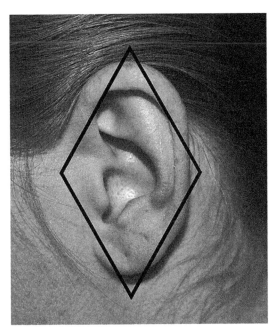

Fig. 2. A field block of the auricle can be achieved with infiltration of local anesthetic in a diamond-shaped formation around the auricle using 4 passes.

Concha and External Auditory Canal

Indications for local anesthesia of the concha and external auditory canal (EAC) include removal of foreign bodies, debridement and cleaning for otitis externa, and cleaning of severe cerumen impaction. Sensory innervation to the concha and the posteroinferior quadrant of the EAC is supplied by the auricular branch of the vagus nerve, whereas the remainder of the EAC is supplied by the auriculotemporal nerve. Several techniques can be used to achieve local anesthesia of the concha and EAC. The most commonly used technique involves a 4-quadrant subcutaneous field block in the lateral portion of the cartilaginous EAC (**Fig. 3**); however, this technique can be extremely painful during administration of the local anesthetic into the sensitive EAC skin. Alternatively, a series of injections can be given anterior to the tragus, along the helical root, and just lateral to the EAC in the concha to achieve the desired effect (**Fig. 4**).[6]

Tympanic Membrane

Indications for local anesthesia of the tympanic membrane (TM) include tympanocentesis; myringotomy; transtympanic injection of gentamicin or steroids; and pressure-equalizing tube placement, removal, or manipulation. A 4-quadrant block of the EAC as described previously is also effective in providing anesthesia of the TM; however, topical anesthesia is generally preferred over the 4-quadrant block because of the painful nature of the 4-quadrant block.

Topical anesthesia

Topical anesthesia of the TM was first reported by Zaufel in 1884 using 10% cocaine dissolved in alcohol.[7] Currently, the most frequently used agent is topical 80% to 90%

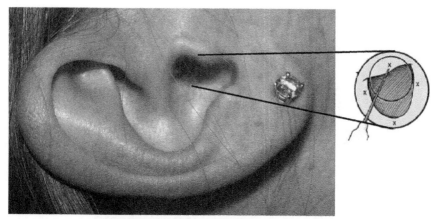

Fig. 3. A 4-quadrant field block of the external auditory canal is performed with subcutaneous injection of local anesthetic until a small elevation of tissue is seen in the lateral canal. An ear speculum is often useful in guiding these injections.

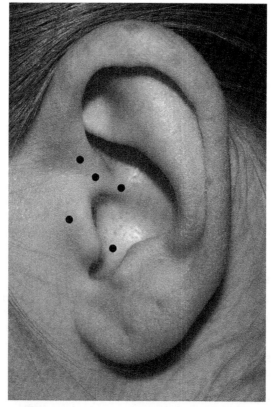

Fig. 4. A series of injections anterior to the tragus, along the helical root, and lateral to the EAC in the concha can also be used to anesthetize the external auditory canal.

liquefied phenol, an effective analgesic agent causing full-thickness analgesia with an immediate effect.[8] The phenol is applied to the TM with an applicator causing the TM to blanch on contact; however, care must be taken to avoid application of phenol to the EAC because of the possibility of systemic absorption through the skin resulting in toxicity, and the possibility of a chemical otitis externa. Another topical agent commonly used for TM anesthesia is a solution of 8% tetracaine base in 70% iso-propyl alcohol. To provide adequate anesthesia for intraoffice procedures, 5 to 10 drops of this solution may be used to fill one-third of the EAC and make contact with the TM for approximately 15 minutes.[9,10] Alternatively, lidocaine and prilocaine in a eutectic mixture of local anesthetics (EMLA) may be applied to the TM using cotton pledgets for approximately 30 to 60 minutes.[11–13] However, this time-consuming procedure has shown mixed results when efficacy has been compared with other topical anesthetic techniques.[13,14]

Transtympanic iontophoresis
Iontophoresis, a procedure in which charged molecules or ions are induced to migrate through tissues under the influence of a direct electrical current, has also been described as a method of achieving anesthesia of the TM using lidocaine or lignocaine (**Fig. 5**).[15,16] However, this technique is not commonly used in a typical practice because of its cumbersome and time-consuming nature, as well as reports that the total anesthetic effect of iontophoresis on the TM may be unpredictable and inade-quate.[17] The first step in transtympanic iontophoresis is to fill the EAC with local anes-thetic warmed to body temperature. Next, a negative electrode is applied to the patient's skin while a positive electrode is placed into the anesthetic solution in the patient's external canal. A current is then applied (ie, gradual increase to a maximum of 0.5 mA at 18 V) for approximately 10 minutes, after which the current is gradually decreased and the anesthetic is suctioned from the EAC.[18]

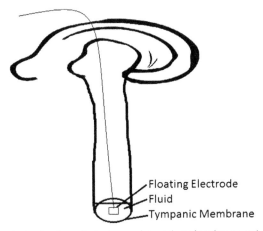

Floating Electrode
Fluid
Tympanic Membrane

Fig. 5. Transtympanic iontophoresis induces charged molecules to migrate through the tympanic membrane tissue under the influence of a direct electrical current. The external canal is filled with the local anesthetic and an electrode is placed into the anesthetic solu-tion to provide the necessary current.

NOSE

Indications for local anesthesia of the nasal cavity include examination using rigid or flexible endoscopes, nasal debridement, control of epistaxis, treatment of nasal fractures, and management of abscesses and hematomas. Both local and topical anesthetic techniques can be used for these purposes, either alone or in conjunction, and have proven to be very effective. For example, when compared with general anesthesia, the selection of one of these anesthetic methods has been shown to have no effect on the results of closed reduction of nasal fractures.[19–21]

Topical Anesthesia

Topical anesthetics, such as lidocaine or pontocaine, are commonly administered in conjunction with a vasoconstricting substance (for decongestion of mucosal edema), such as 0.05% oxymetazoline, before examination or treatment of the nasal cavity by the otorhinolaryngologist. This solution can be sprayed in the nasal cavity via atomizer or applied to cotton pledgets, which are then placed in the nasal cavity with bayonet forceps to cover branches of the anterior and posterior ethmoid, sphenopalatine, and nasopalatine nerves, along the nasal septum and lateral nasal wall. Alternatively, cocaine is a rapidly effective and powerful topical anesthetic and vasoconstricting agent when applied to the nasal mucosa on cotton pledgets. It is available in solution preparations ranging from 2% to 10%, with 4 mL of 4% solution being the most frequently used preparation. When using cocaine for topical anesthesia of the nasal cavity, the treating physician should keep in mind the reported maximum dosage of 200 mg or 2 to 3 mg/kg, and consider using cardiopulmonary monitoring. Studies have shown that only approximately one third of cocaine solution placed on pledgets is absorbed via the nasal mucosa, although longer application times most likely result in increased absorption.[22] The clinical use of cocaine in otorhinolaryngology has decreased significantly in the past 25 years, and may reflect a better understanding of its potential toxicities and the availability of safer alternative medications.[23]

Local Anesthesia

Sufficient anesthesia of the internal nasal cavity can be achieved by injection of local anesthetic agents, such as lidocaine, along the nasal septum and lateral walls and floor of the nasal cavity. The external nasal nerve (also termed the external branch of the anterior ethmoidal nerve) can be blocked with an intercartilaginous injection of the nasal dorsum from the region of the rhinion to the supratip region (**Fig. 6**). A nasopalatine nerve block can be achieved with an injection at the base of the columella and nasal tip just inside of the nasal sill.

An infraorbital nerve block can be achieved via an intranasal, intraoral, or transcutaneous approach and injection in the region of the infraorbital foramen. Vasoconstrictors should not be used to avoid vasoconstriction of the facial artery, which may lie on either side of the needle. The infraorbital foramen can be difficult to palpate externally, but can be found on the inferior border of the infraorbital rim, in line with the pupil when the patient is looking straight ahead (see **Fig. 6**). This is the site of injection when using the transcutaneous approach. The transnasal approach is performed with an injection that passes through the vestibule into the facial soft tissues, just below the mid-orbital rim in the region of the infraorbital foramen. Alternatively, for the intraoral approach, the gingivobuccal sulcus above the first premolar is anesthetized with topical anesthetic, as described in the following section about the oral cavity. Next, while keeping a palpating finger in place over the infraorbital rim, a needle is introduced into this space and advanced approximately 2 cm toward the infraorbital foramen (although

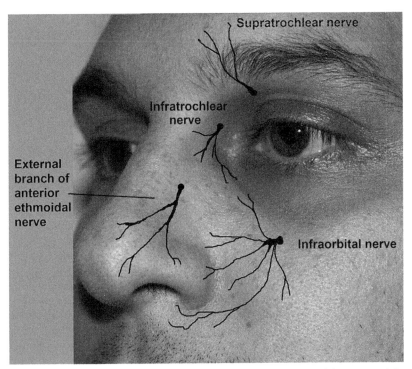

Fig. 6. Sensory innervation of the external nose includes the supratrochlear nerve, infratrochlear nerve, infraorbital nerve, and external branch of the anterior ethmoidal nerve.

this distance varies from patient to patient), and local anesthetic is injected in the region of the infraorbital foramen. Care should be taken to ensure that the needle is not advanced too far posteriorly and superiorly when performing this intraoral injection, so that the orbit is not entered inadvertently. Although the level of anesthesia achieved by these 3 approaches is comparable, one study found that the duration of anesthesia was prolonged significantly via the intraoral approach.[24]

ORAL CAVITY AND OROPHARYNX

Indications for local anesthesia of the oral cavity and oropharynx include examination and treatment of the teeth, closure of a laceration, incision and drainage of a peritonsillar abscess, and treatment of patients who have sustained severe dentoalveolar trauma (ie, maxillomandibular fixation for mandible fractures).

Topical Anesthesia

The use of topical anesthetics applied to the mucous membranes in the oral cavity is useful in alleviating the pain associated with infiltration of local anesthetics, which can be a source of great apprehension for many patients. To minimize the amount of anesthetic that is swept away by saliva, the area to be anesthetized is first dried thoroughly. The physician's anesthetic of choice (ie, 20% benzocaine, or 10% lidocaine) is then applied to the area that is to be anesthetized with gentle pressure for a few minutes using a cotton-tip applicator. Once the topical anesthetic has taken effect, the physician may proceed with the desired procedure, although injection of local anesthetic is typically required for adequate anesthesia.

Topical anesthesia of the oropharynx can be achieved with an anesthetic spray, such as 20% benzocaine, or by asking the patient to gargle a viscous local anesthetic, such as 2% viscous lidocaine. It is important for the physician to keep in mind that topical benzocaine has been reported to rarely cause methemoglobinemia, a potentially life-threatening medical condition, with incidence rates ranging from 0.04% to 0.30%.[25–28] Clinically, acquired methemoglobinemia is characterized by cyanosis, low pulse oximetric readings, and chocolate-brown blood on arterial blood gas sampling with normal arterial pO_2 values. Diagnosis is confirmed by measurement of elevated methemoglobin levels on arterial blood sampling, and treatment includes intravenous administration of the antidote, methylene blue. If an invasive procedure, such as incision and drainage of a peritonsillar abscess, is to be performed, topical anesthesia may be followed by submucosal injection of local anesthetic, such as 1% lidocaine, in the desired location.

Local Anesthesia

If anesthesia of an individual tooth is desired, a slow supraperiosteal injection of local anesthetic can be administered in the area of the corresponding tooth root with the bevel of the needle facing the bone. The objective is to place the anesthetic in proximity to the supporting bony structures to achieve penetration of the anesthetic into the cortex of bone, and subsequently to reach the nerve. The palatal side of the tooth can also be injected if the desired level of anesthesia is not reached. Regional nerve blocks can be achieved using the same technique in the region of specific teeth (**Fig. 7**). The posterior alveolar nerve (supplying sensory innervation to the ipsilateral maxillary molar teeth) can be anesthetized with an injection in the region of the distal buccal root of the upper second molar with the needle directed toward the maxillary tuberosity, and then along the curvature of the maxillary tuberosity to a depth of approximately 2 cm. The middle superior alveolar nerve (supplying sensory innervation to the mesiobuccal root of the maxillary first molar and the ipsilateral premolars) can be anesthetized with an injection between the second premolar and first molar. The anterior

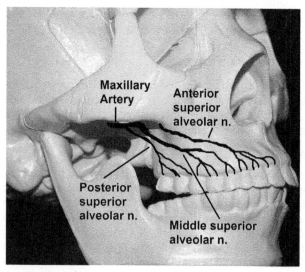

Fig. 7. Sensory innervation of the maxillary dentition is provided by the posterior, middle, and anterior superior alveolar nerves.

superior alveolar nerve (supplying sensory innervation to the ipsilateral canine and incisors) can be anesthetized with an injection placed at the apex of the canine tooth. Alternatively, an infraorbital nerve block (described previously in the section on anesthesia of the nose), anesthetizes the anterior and middle superior alveolar nerves, in addition to the skin of the upper lip, the skin of the nose, and the lower eyelid.

An inferior alveolar nerve block provides anesthesia to all of the teeth of the ipsilateral mandible and desensitizes the lower lip and the chin via block of the mental nerve. To perform this block, the pterygomandibular triangle is first visualized and topically anesthetized by placing a thumb in the mouth and an index finger externally behind the ramus to retract the tissues. Once topical anesthesia of this area has been obtained, local anesthetic is introduced through the mucosa of the pterygomandibular triangle approximately 1 cm above the occlusal surface of the molars, and is advanced until it has reached the bone where the anesthetic agent is injected (**Fig. 8**). When performing this injection, the angle of entry is of great importance, as directing the needle too far posteriorly may result in temporary facial paralysis as a result of injection into the parotid tissue. To achieve the appropriate angle, the syringe should be held parallel to the occlusal surfaces of the teeth and angled so that the barrel of the syringe lies between the first and the second premolars on the contralateral side of the mandible. When a block of the inferior alveolar nerve is performed, the nearby lingual nerve is often blocked as well, resulting in anesthesia of the anterior two-thirds of the tongue. Thus, the same technique can be used if anesthesia of the tongue is desired for a procedure such as a lingual biopsy.

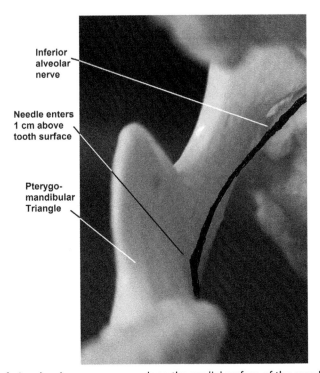

Fig. 8. The inferior alveolar nerve courses along the medial surface of the mandibular ramus where a block can be performed by injecting local anesthetic in the region of the pterygomandibular triangle.

If anesthesia of only the ipsilateral lower lip is desired, an isolated mental nerve block can be achieved by infiltration of local anesthetic around the mental foramen. This can be accomplished via an intraoral or an extraoral approach, although the intraoral technique has been shown to be less painful.[29] The mental foramen is identified by palpation about 1 cm inferior and anterior to the second premolar, roughly in line with the pupil when the patient is looking straight ahead. When using the intraoral approach, the lower labial fold adjacent to the first or second premolar is topically anesthetized, and the injection is directed toward the mental foramen.

LARYNX

Indications for local anesthesia of the larynx include diagnostic laryngoscopy and bronchoscopy, transnasal esophagoscopy, and placement of an endotracheal tube when awake endotracheal intubation is indicated either electively or emergently.

Topical Anesthesia

Topical anesthesia of the oropharyngeal and nasal mucosa can be helpful when performing endoscopic procedures. Techniques for topical anesthesia of the nasal mucosa and oropharyngeal mucosa were previously described in this text. In the nasal cavity, this includes application of a topical anesthetic, typically used in conjunction with a vasoconstricting substance, in the form of a spray via atomizer or application using cotton pledgets. Benzocaine 20% spray or 2% viscous lidocaine can similarly be used to anesthetize the oropharyngeal mucosa. To anesthetize the vocal cords, the patient may be asked to inspire deeply while topical anesthetic is sprayed into the nasal cavity. Alternatively, transnasal esophagoscopes can be used to apply 4% lidocaine directly to the larynx through the irrigation port on the endoscope.

Local Anesthesia

A superior laryngeal nerve block can be used to anesthetize the supraglottic larynx by effectively blocking the internal branch of the superior laryngeal nerve, which supplies sensory input from the inferior aspect of the epiglottis down to the vocal cords. To perform a superior laryngeal nerve block, the patient's neck is extended and the hyoid bone is displaced laterally toward the side to be blocked. A small-gauge needle, such as a 27-gauge needle, is advanced approximately 3 mm inferior to the greater cornu of

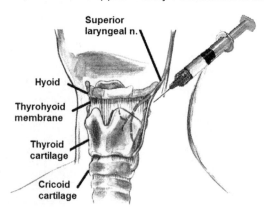

Fig. 9. A superior laryngeal nerve block can be performed by injecting local anesthetic medial and lateral to the thyrohyoid membrane at a level just inferior to the greater cornu of the hyoid bone, providing anesthesia to the supraglottic larynx.

the hyoid bone until it passes through the thyrohyoid membrane, at which point a slight loss of resistance is felt (**Fig. 9**). Once this has been accomplished, 3 mL of local anesthetic solution is injected superficial and deep to the thyrohyoid membrane.

If anesthesia of the subglottis and trachea is desired, a translaryngeal block can be performed by locating the cricothyroid membrane and introducing a small-caliber needle in the midline. Once confirmation of correct placement is established by aspiration of air, 5 mL of 4% lidocaine can be injected rapidly. This will usually result in stimulation of a forceful cough reflex, which aids in distributing the topical anesthetic within the subglottis and trachea.

SUMMARY

Topical and local anesthetic techniques have long been used safely by otorhinolaryngologists for office procedures. There are numerous advantages to using these techniques, including reduced cost of procedures and postprocedure care, faster recovery times, and the maintenance of a conscious patient with the ability to maintain his or her own airway, contain his or her own gastric secretions, and communicate with the treating physician. Using various techniques in topical application and injection of local anesthetics, numerous procedures can be performed safely on the external face, ear, nose, oral cavity, nasopharynx, oropharynx, hypopharynx, and larynx.

REFERENCES

1. Apostolopoulos K, Labropoulou E, Samaan R, et al. Ropivacaine compared to lidocaine for tonsillectomy under local anaesthesia. Eur Arch Otorhinolaryngol 2003;260(7):355–7.
2. Bredenkamp JK, Abemayor E, Wackym PA, et al. Tonsillectomy under local anesthesia: a safe and effective alternative. Am J Otolaryngol 1990;11(1):18–22.
3. Metzinger SE, Bailey DJ, Boyce RG, et al. Local anesthesia in rhinoplasty: a new twist? Ear Nose Throat J 1992;71(9):405–6.
4. Arndt KA, Burton C, Noe J. Minimizing the pain of local anesthesia. Plast Reconstr Surg 1983;72(5):676–9.
5. Häfner HM, Röcken M, Breuninger H. Epinephrine-supplemented local anesthetics for ear and nose surgery: clinical use without complications in more than 10,000 surgical procedures. J Dtsch Dermatol Ges 2005;3(3):195–9.
6. Riviello RJ, Brown NA. Otolaryngologic procedures. In: Roberts JR, Hedges JR, editors. Clinical procedures in emergency medicine. 5th edition. Philadelphia: WB Saunders; 2010. Chapter 64.
7. Hirsch C. Anaesthesia of the external ear. Acta Otolaryngol 1934;21:256–78.
8. Weisskopf A. Phenol anesthesia for myringotomy. Laryngoscope 1983;93:114.
9. Carrasco VN, Prazma T, Biggers P. A safe effective anesthetic technique for outpatient myringotomy tube placement. Laryngoscope 1993;103:92–3.
10. Hoffman RA, Li CL. Tetracaine topical anesthesia for myringotomy. Laryngoscope 2001;111(9):1636–8.
11. Timms MS, O'Malley S, Keith AO. Experience with a new topical anaesthetic in otology. Clin Otolaryngol Allied Sci 1988;13(6):485–90.
12. Whittet HB, Williams HO, Wright A. An evaluation of topical anaesthesia for myringotomy. Clin Otolaryngol Allied Sci 1988;13(6):481–4.
13. Luotonen J, Laitakari K, Karjalainen H, et al. EMLA in local anaesthesia of the tympanic membrane. Acta Otolaryngol Suppl 1992;492:63–7.

14. Jyväkorpi M. A comparison of topical Emla cream with Bonain's solution for anesthesia of the tympanic membrane during tympanocentesis. Eur Arch Otorhinolaryngol 1996;253(4–5):234–6.
15. Comeau M, Brummett R, Vernon J. Local anesthesia of the ear by iontophoresis. Arch Otolaryngol 1973;98(2):114–20.
16. Hasegawa M, Saito Y, Watanabe I. Iontophoretic anaesthesia of the tympanic membrane. Clin Otolaryngol Allied Sci 1978;3(1):63–6.
17. Johannessen J, Hvidegaard T, Brask T. The influence of lidocaine and iontophoresis on the pain threshold of the human eardrum. Arch Otolaryngol 1982;108(4): 201–3.
18. Sirimanna KS, Madden GJ, Miles S. Anaesthesia of the tympanic membrane: comparison of EMLA cream and iontophoresis. J Laryngol Otol 1990;104(3): 195–6.
19. Cook JA, McRae RD, Irving RM, et al. A randomized comparison of manipulation of the fractured nose under local and general anaesthesia. Clin Otolaryngol Allied Sci 1990;15(4):343–6.
20. Waldron J, Mitchell DB, Ford G. Reduction of fractured nasal bones: local versus general anaesthesia. Clin Otolaryngol Allied Sci 1989;14(4):357–9.
21. Atighechi S, Baradaranfar MH, Akbari SA. Reduction of nasal bone fractures: a comparative study of general, local, and topical anesthesia techniques. J Craniofac Surg 2009;20(2):382–4.
22. Greinwald JH Jr, Holtel MR. Absorption of topical cocaine in rhinologic procedures. Laryngoscope 1996;106(10):1223–5.
23. Long H, Greller H, Mercurio-Zappala M, et al. Medicinal use of cocaine: a shifting paradigm over 25 years. Laryngoscope 2004;114(9):1625–9.
24. Lynch MT, Syverud SA, Schwab RA, et al. Comparison of intraoral and percutaneous approaches for infraorbital nerve block. Acad Emerg Med 1994;1:514.
25. Kane GC, Hoehn SM, Behrenbeck TR, et al. Benzocaine-induced methemoglobinemia based on the Mayo Clinic experience from 28 478 transesophageal echocardiograms: incidence, outcomes, and predisposing factors. Arch Intern Med 2007;167(18):1977–82.
26. Novaro GM, Aronow HD, Militello MA, et al. Benzocaine-induced methemoglobinemia: experience from a high-volume transesophageal echocardiography laboratory. J Am Soc Echocardiogr 2003;16(2):170–5.
27. Aepfelbacher FC, Breen P, Manning WJ. Methemoglobinemia and topical pharyngeal anesthesia. N Engl J Med 2003;348(1):85–6.
28. Bheemreddy S, Messineo F, Roychoudhury D. Methemoglobinemia following transesophageal echocardiography: a case report and review. Echocardiography 2006;23(4):319–21.
29. Syverud SA, Jenkins JM, Schwab RA, et al. A comparative study of the percutaneous versus intraoral technique for mental nerve block. Acad Emerg Med 1994; 1:509.

Laryngeal Mask Airways in Ear, Nose, and Throat Procedures

Jeff E. Mandel, MD, MS

KEYWORDS

- Laryngeal masks • Otorhinolaryngology • Tracheostomy
- Thyroidectomy • Adenotonsillectomy
- Endoscopic sinus surgery • Laryngeal framework surgery

The laryngeal mask airway (LMA) was developed by Archie Brain and introduced into clinical practice in 1988. Numerous variants of the LMA have been developed by Brain and others over the ensuing years. Important differences can be found among these devices, and although the term *LMA* is a trademark of the Laryngeal Mask Company, many of the techniques described herein are likely applicable to competitors of the LMA. The makers of these devices have shown substantial equivalence to the LMA for the U.S. Food and Drug Administration. Individual readers must decide whether these products are adequate substitutes for the techniques described with the predicate device.

The LMA has developed a considerable following because of its lack of tracheal stimulation, which can be a considerable advantage in ear, nose, and throat (ENT) procedures. The incidence of coughing on emergence has been shown to be lower with the LMA than with the endotracheal tube (ETT).[1] Although other approaches to smooth emergence have been described, few would argue that it is as easy to achieve a smooth emergence with an ETT as with an LMA.

Another advantage of the LMA is the ability to insert the device without the use of neuromuscular blocking agents (NMBs). Although many practitioners routinely intubate without NMBs, the practice is not without critics, and few would argue that NMBs should be routinely used in placing the LMA. Avoidance of muscle relaxants in ENT procedures may be advantageous, particularly in outpatient settings.

A frequent comorbidity in ENT surgery is recurrent upper respiratory infections (URIs), particularly in children undergoing adenotonsillectomy. Tait and colleagues[2] reported a prospective comparison of ETT and LMA in 82 children undergoing a range of procedures who presented with an active URI. Children anesthetized through LMA

Department of Anesthesiology and Critical Care, University of Pennsylvania School of Medicine, 3400 Spruce Street, Philadelphia, PA 19104, USA
E-mail address: mandelj@uphs.upenn.edu

Anesthesiology Clin 28 (2010) 469–483
doi:10.1016/j.anclin.2010.07.005   **anesthesiology.theclinics.com**

were significantly less likely to experience bronchospasm, coughing, and oxygen desaturation. Although in a retrospective review of 831 children managed with LMA von Ungern-Sternberg and colleagues[3] found that recent URIs doubled the risk of these complications, this risk was significantly less than the 11-fold increase associated with ETT.

ENT procedures often cause bleeding in the pharynx. Endotracheal intubation is associated with prolonged diminution of laryngeal protective reflexes.[4] In a prospective study comparing laryngeal responses during general anesthesia in 20 patients randomized to either ETT or LMA, Tanaka and colleagues[5] found a greater attenuation in the laryngeal response and a greater narrowing of the vocal cord opening in patients with the ETT.

Another advantage of the LMA is its utility in airway rescue. Although LMA is certainly contraindicated in some patients with laryngeal pathology, the LMA is often the airway of first resort when dealing with patients with pharyngeal pathology.

Indications for LMA that apply to specific situations in ENT surgery can be divided into several areas:

A conduit for surgical access to the glottis and trachea
An aid to neurologic monitoring
A means to isolate the glottis from bleeding from pharyngeal sources.

When considering the range of procedures in ENT surgery, the advantages of the LMA in appropriate settings will become increasingly apparent.

LMA FOR OTOLOGY

Otologic procedures present several challenges for anesthetists. Access to the airway is often limited, and head movement from mask ventilation may interfere with the procedure. Although some procedures may be performed with sedation, airway obstruction may be difficult to manage. Coughing and straining on emergence may place patients at risk for complications, such as hematoma and cerebrospinal fluid otorrhea. The LMA offers an attractive alternative for airway management.

Duff[6] reviewed 100 consecutive cases in which the LMA was used for otologic procedures. All procedures were performed with the table turned 180° away from the anesthetist. Patients included 49 children and 51 adults. Children were anesthetized with nitrous oxide and isoflurane; adults with propofol, fentanyl, and inhalational anesthesia. In one patient, surgery was interrupted for 3 minutes because of patient movement. In the 73 patients in whom the head was moved for application of a head dressing, no coughing was observed.

Ayala and colleagues[7] reviewed 484 cases over a 3-year period, of which 35% were managed with LMA and 65% with ETT. Induction and emergence times in the LMA group were shorter by 2.6 and 2.2 minutes, respectively. Three patients in the LMA group were converted to ETT because of excessive leak.

In the author's experience when using the LMA in otology, spontaneous ventilation may result in a rocky respiratory pattern from abdominal breathing, and phonation from adduction of the vocal cords during early inspiration. These factors may be overcome by using pressure-cycled ventilation and total intravenous anesthesia, providing surgeons with a more tranquil field while permitting emergence without coughing or straining.

LMA FOR RHINOLOGY

Use of the LMA in functional endoscopic sinus surgery (FESS) may seem counterintuitive to the uninitiated. Limited access to the airway and the potential for blood in the pharynx would seem to preclude the use of supraglottic airways. Although these issues cannot be ignored, several published reports have addressed these concerns.

In a 1992 retrospective review of 103 cases of minor nasal surgery (polypectomies and antral washouts), Daum and O'Reilly[8] found no evidence of airway contamination. Two patients were "known difficult intubations" and were managed without difficulty. The authors noted that the ability to perform brief procedures without the use of suxamethonium was advantageous in avoiding myalgias.

Interest in the use of the LMA in ENT increased after the introduction of the flexible LMA (fLMA), depicted in **Fig. 1**. Williams and colleagues[9] prospectively compared ETT and fLMA in 66 patients undergoing sinus surgery. A throat pack was placed in all patients, and was removed at the end of surgery. After removal of the throat pack and suctioning, the ETT was immediately removed and a Guedel airway was placed while the patients were deeply anesthetized, whereas the fLMAs were removed when the patients were awake. Airway maintenance was considered to be uniformly easy in the fLMA group, whereas 34.5% of patients required jaw thrust to maintain a patent airway after removal of the ETT. Before removal, a fiberoptic bronchoscope was placed to assess the airway; blood was seen in the larynx of two patients with the fLMA and in the trachea of three patients with the ETT. Laryngospasm was seen in one patient in the ETT group, and none in the fLMA group. The authors concluded that the fLMA could protect the airway from bleeding during sinus surgery, and provided a more stable airway than deep extubation.

Webster and colleagues[10] prospectively compared fLMA with ETT in 114 patients undergoing intranasal surgery. Patients were allocated to three groups: fLMA removed awake, ETT removed awake, and ETT removed deep. Airway examination for contamination with blood was equivalent among the groups, whereas incidence of laryngospasm was significantly greater in the ETT + deep extubation group, and the incidence of low saturation on postanesthesia care unit admission was higher in the ETT + awake extubation group. Coughing was less frequent and less severe in the fLMA group. The authors concluded that the fLMA offered advantages compared with ETT removed either under deep anesthesia or awake.

In a prospective observational study of 200 patients undergoing intranasal surgery, Ahmed and Vohra[11] assessed soiling of the glottic aspect of the fLMA. In 87% of cases, blood was excluded from the fLMA, whereas in 11%, minor soiling of the cuff was seen. In only 2% of cases was blood seen in the bowl of the fLMA, and blood was never observed in the tube. No patients exhibited clinical signs of aspiration. The authors concluded that the fLMA was effective in protecting the airway until the patient was awake.

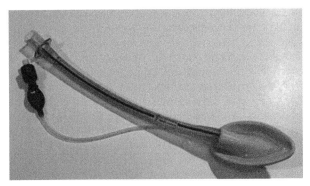

Fig. 1. The flexible laryngeal mask airway.

In a nonrandomized, prospective comparison of ETT and fLMA in patients under-going intranasal surgery, Kaplan and colleagues[12] performed fiberoptic inspection of 31 ETTs and 43 fLMAs. They found that blood staining of any portion of the airway was significantly higher with ETT (84.8% vs 19.5%), but blood distal to the tip of the airway device was more common with fLMA (14.6% vs 3.2%). The authors noted that blood was frequently seen pooling above the cuff of the ETT in the subglottic trachea, and attributed a trend toward poorer emergence in this group to the greater frequency of blood in contact with the vocal cords. They concluded that the fLMA provided more comprehensive protection of the glottis from blood, diverting it away from the glottis to the piriform sinuses, where it could be suctioned at the end of the procedure.

Atef and Fawaz[13] randomized 60 patients to fLMA or ETT and compared blood loss, visualization conditions, and the rate of remifentanil infusion required to maintain systolic blood pressure near 80 mm Hg. Blood loss was significantly less in the fLMA group (200 vs 299 mL). Visualization conditions were assessed at 15-minute intervals by a single surgeon using a six-point scale; scores were better in the fLMA group for the first 15 minutes of surgery, but equivalent thereafter. Remifentanil infu-sion rate was titrated to maintain systolic blood pressure at less than 80 mm Hg; the fLMA group required a lower rate (0.3 vs 0.44 µg/kg/min). Heart rate and mean blood pressure were also lower during the first 15 minutes of the procedure in the fLMA group, which likely explained the better visualization conditions during that period. The investigators noted that the stress response to intubation was the likely reason for the initial higher blood pressure and heart rate, and although this could be overcome with higher remifentanil infusion rates, the fLMA provided excellent visu-alization conditions at lower infusion rates.

In a randomized study of 60 children aged 1 to 12 years, Al-Mazrou and colleagues[14] compared uncuffed ETT with gauze throat packing and LMA for intra-nasal procedures. Contamination of the glottis and trachea was equivalent between groups, although soiling of the interior was less with the LMA. No adverse events were noted, and the authors concluded that the LMA provided protection equivalent to the uncuffed ETT in this age group.

The use of the LMA for intranasal surgery is supported by five prospective studies and two observational studies. In almost 500 cases included in these reports, no serious adverse events were described and no case reports of serious adverse events attribut-able to use of the LMA in intranasal surgery were found. The ability of the fLMA to provide a wakeup with fewer episodes of coughing and laryngospasm is well established.

Clearly, some patients are not candidates for the LMA, and an adequate seal cannot be obtained in all patients. For those contemplating adopting the technique, several points should be observed. First, placement of the flexible LMA requires more atten-tion to technique than the conventional LMA. Second, proper sizing and positioning are important, and using fiberoptic laryngoscopy to confirm placement is helpful whenever possible and should be performed routinely during the first 20 cases. Third, determination of the leak pressure should be performed routinely through assessing the pressure achieved by closing the adjustable pressure limiting valve at 2 liters per minute of fresh gas flow. Only when the pressure exceeds 15 cm H_2O should the glottis considered to have adequate protection. Fourth, when positive pressure ventilation is used, pressure-cycled ventilation below the leak pressure is essential to avoid bubbles of blood and saliva interfering with visualization. Fifth, the anesthesia circuit should not be tethered to the chest, because extension of the neck may displace the LMA. When observing these simple measures, most problems can be avoided.

Although many practitioners feel most comfortable using spontaneous ventilation with an LMA, the author uses pressure-controlled ventilation at pressures below the leak pressure, particularly when using total intravenous anesthesia. Consideration should be given to the oxygen concentration delivered when electrocautery is used, because a sizeable leak can increase the risk of a fire.

LMA for Adenotonsillectomy

Several factors motivate the use of the LMA in adenotonsillectomy. The LMA is typically placed without neuromuscular blocking agents, which may result in faster emergence in short procedures. In children requiring inhalational induction, the LMA can be placed at a lighter plane of anesthesia, freeing the anesthetist to perform intravenous cannulation. The LMA can remain in place until emergence, protecting the glottis from blood and secretions. The LMA is less stimulating to the trachea, which may be advantageous in children with tonsillitis who have chronic upper respiratory infections. Several prospective studies have examined these issues.

Williams and Bailey[15] reported a prospective comparison of fLMA and ETT in 104 children undergoing adenotonsillectomy. Although four patients were withdrawn from the fLMA arm, two because of inability to place the LMA and two because of obstruction by the Boyle-Davis (B-D) mouth gag, patients in the LMA group had significantly fewer airway complications attributable to blood aspiration on emergence. In a prospective comparison of fLMA and ETT in 99 children undergoing adenotonsillectomy, Webster and colleagues[16] found a higher rate of obstruction with the B-D mouth gag than Williams and Bailey, but found similar rates of postoperative airway complications between groups. In 19 of the patients in the fLMA group, fiberoptic assessment of the airway was performed and no evidence was seen of blood in the airway. Additionally, in no instances was blood found in the bowl of the LMA.

These reports triggered some controversy. In a letter to the *British Journal of Anaesthesia*, Heath and Sinnathamby[17] noted that in the initial experience of 112 children managed with the fLMA at Lewisham Hospital in London, problems with obstruction were observed in 20.5% of cases, and kinking of the flexible tube in the B-D mouth gag was seen as the cause in "virtually every instance." In reply, Williams and Bailey[18] noted that at the Royal National Throat, Nose and Ear Hospital, the fLMA was used in more than 50% of the 1302 adenotonsillectomies performed in the preceding 12 months with "no major problems."

A question not addressed by the earlier studies was the ability to obtain a complete resection. In a prospective comparison of fLMA and ETT in 91 patients, Hern and colleagues[19] found significantly better visualization conditions and resection tissue weight with ETT, and noted an 11.4% rate of having to convert from fLMA to ETT because of inadequate access or problems with ventilation.

Concerns over the effect of changes in head position and use of the B-D mouth gag on pharyngeal seal were addressed in studies by Keller and Brimacombe[20] and Brimacombe and colleagues.[21] In a randomized crossover study of 20 paralyzed adults, minimal differences were observed in leak pressure between the standard and flexible LMA, with lower leak pressures in flexion. In a study in fresh cadavers, the B-D mouth gag was found not to influence leak pressure. Additionally, the pressure associated with passage of water placed in the mouth into the trachea was determined. When the leak pressure equaled 12 cm H_2O, aspiration was observed in 5% of cadavers. The investigators recommended routine assessment of leak pressure to exceed 15 cm H_2O to provide adequate protection from aspiration.

In a review of prospectively collected data from 1126 children undergoing tonsillectomy and/or adenoidectomy with the fLMA, Gravningsbråten and colleagues[22] found a 0.6% rate of conversion to ETT, with all failures caused by unacceptable leak pressures. Kretz and colleagues[23] reviewed the experience over 4 years and 2898 adenotonsillectomies at the Olga Hospital in Stuttgart and found increasing use of the LMA over this period, from 0 per 749 procedures in 1994 to 1026 per 1160 in 1997. The LMA permitted greater procedural efficiency and a lower rate of laryngospasm and obstruction.

Several postal surveys of LMA use in adenotonsillectomy have been conducted. Hatcher and Stack[24] surveyed consultant anesthesiologists with an interest in ENT in three National Health Service districts. Of 110 questionnaires mailed, 88 were returned. Of these, 14 respondents used the LMA routinely in adenotonsillectomy, although of the 39 who responded that they had used the LMA on more than one occasion, 13 reported that they had experienced difficulty associated with its use. Ecoffey and colleagues,[25] working with data from the French National Survey of Anesthesia performed in 1996, excerpted 653 cases of tonsillectomy in children younger than 15 years. Of these cases, 64% were performed with the ETT, 2% with the LMA, and 34% with natural airways. No distinction was made between outcomes with ETT and LMA, although cases performed with natural airways were typically short procedures in healthy children.

Clarke and colleagues[26] mailed questionnaires to all 305 Royal College Tutors in the United Kingdom, with instructions for those who did not perform anesthesia for ENT procedures to forward the questionnaire to a colleague who did. Of the 272 hospitals responding that they performed ENT procedures, the ETT was used in 87% of children aged 0 to 3 years, 79% of children aged 3 to 16 years, and 73% of adults undergoing tonsillectomy, with the remainder using either a single-use or a reusable LMA. The purpose of the study was to measure compliance with guidelines intended to avoid the spread of variant Creutzfeldt-Jacob disease (also known as Bovine Spongiform Encephalitis), and did not include questions on relative rates of success with ETT versus LMA.

Allford and Guruswamy[27] sent questionnaires to all Royal College Tutors, soliciting answers from those who specialized in pediatric ENT procedures. Of the 173 responses, 79% preferred endotracheal intubation. Again, no questions were directed at relative success of the techniques. Respondents did note a significant preference for intravenous induction, and used NMBs in fewer than 50% of intubations.

Using the LMA for adenotonsillectomy may have advantages, particularly in the hands of experienced practitioners. It is certainly used by a significant minority of British anesthetists. It may reduce the rate of airway complications in patients presenting with a URI. Although using the LMA may have advantages in patients undergoing inhalational induction before intravenous access, and in avoiding the use of NMBs, these practices seem to be less prevalent. With careful positioning of the B-D mouth gag, kinking should be a rare occurrence. However, when complications occur with the LMA in adenotonsillectomy, it tends to be abandoned in favor of the ETT, although the converse is rarely the case. Practitioners should weigh the evidence and decide whether they possess the perseverance to adopt this technique.

LMA for Percutaneous Tracheostomy

The first reports of LMA as a means of airway control during percutaneous dilational tracheostomy (PDT) were presented by Dexter[28] and Tarpey and colleagues,[29] who almost simultaneously reported cases in which the LMA was used to facilitate the procedure. Further cases were reported by Lyons and Flynn.[30] Sustić and colleagues[31] described the use of ultrasound guidance to facilitate this technique in a morbidly obese patient in whom transillumination was unsuccessful in delineating the anatomy.

Systematic investigation of the use of LMA with PDT was first reported by Verghese and colleagues[32] in a prospective observational study of 10 patients. The authors placed an intubating LMA (iLMA) behind the existing ETT, finding adequate conditions in all patients. In a prospective randomized comparison of ETT and LMA for ventilation during PDT in 60 patients, Dosemeci and colleagues[33] found shorter procedure times and lower carbon dioxide elevation with the LMA. No patient in either group exhibited desaturation below 96%, and changes in Pao_2 were minor and not significantly different. In another prospective randomized comparison in 60 patients, Ambesh and colleagues[34] found LMA to be associated with a 33% rate of hypoventilation and gastric distension, although they noted unintended ETT cuff puncture in two patients and ETT impalement in another two. A limitation of this study was the use of size 3 LMAs in women and size 4 LMAs in men, which would account for the greater frequency of leak.

In a prospective observational study of 23 patients undergoing PDT, Craven and colleagues[35] exchanged the ETT for the Proseal LMA (pLMA) and assessed adequacy of ventilation. In 11 patients, no decrement in tidal volume was observed; in 11 patients decrements of less than 100 mL were found; and only one patient showed a decrement of 200 mL. The median value for the lowest arterial saturation across the cohort was 95%.

Linstedt and colleagues[36] noted that damage to the fiberoptic bronchoscope from the tracheal puncture occurred in 1% to 2% of cases in their study. In a prospective observational study of 86 patients, the iLMA was used as the airway after extubation. In one patient, iLMA placement was impossible, and in an additional four, ventilation was judged to be inadequate, requiring reintubation. Visualization of the subglottic trachea was achieved in 90% of patients. Linstedt and colleagues[37] subsequently reported a prospective, randomized comparison of ETT and iLMA for PDT. Visualization of tracheal structures was judged to be "good" or "very good" in 94% of patients in the iLMA group versus 66% of those in the ETT group. Increases in $Paco_2$ were greater in the ETT group (59 vs 51). Two patients in the ETT group experienced unintended extubation during the procedure, and in an additional patient the bronchoscope was damaged during tracheal puncture. One patient in the iLMA group required reintubation because of failure to obtain adequate ventilation.

The use of the LMA as a conduit for ventilation during PDT has significant advantages over withdrawing an ETT into a subglottic position. Familiarity with visualization of glottic structures using flexible bronchoscopy is a skill that can easily be acquired during elective procedures in the operating room, as is the use of the LMA for positive pressure ventilation. Use of the iLMA and pLMA is particularly helpful in this technique. Although the use of the iLMA permits the reintroduction of an ETT should ventilation be inadequate, devices such as the Aintree intubation catheter permit reintubation through the LMA or pLMA.[38]

LMA for Laryngology

Surgical access to the larynx with suspension laryngoscopy or rigid bronchoscopy may be challenging. Although the anesthesiologist is only concerned with securing ventilation, a full view of the vocal cords may be unobtainable in 25% of patients.[39] Obtaining full visualization of the glottis may require extreme measures; removal of the incisors has been reported to permit access to the anterior commissure.[40,41] Suspension laryngoscopy may produce significant hemodynamic responses, and may require use of NMBs to avoid movement. The LMA provides an alternate route to the vocal cords when used in conjunction with the flexible bronchoscope, permitting continual delivery of oxygen and volatile anesthetics during the procedure without impeding access.

In a prospective observational study of 10 patients, Brimacombe and colleagues[42] showed that the vocal cords could be biopsied without significant complications. Kanagalingam and colleagues[43] reported use of potassium titanyl phosphate laser passed through a bronchoscope inserted through an LMA for ablation of lesions of the anterior vocal folds in two patients in whom suspension laryngoscopy had failed. Windfuhr and Remmert[44] reported a case of a 130-kg man with a Mallampati class IV airway examination who required intubation with a Bullard laryngoscope whose lesion was inaccessible with direct laryngoscopy, and who subsequently was unable to tolerate an attempt at sedated fiberoptic resection. After induction of general anesthesia, an iLMA was placed and a fiberoptic bronchoscope passed to obtain a full view of the lesion that was resected with a biopsy forceps and cauterized with argon plasma coagulation.

Chang and colleagues[45] reported an additional case in which iLMA was used to access an anterior lesion inaccessible with suspension laryngoscopy. Chang and colleagues[46] subsequently performed a randomized comparison of the iLMA with suspension laryngoscopy in 40 patients. Percentage of glottic opening was significantly higher in the iLMA group (100% vs 80%), and blood pressure and heart rate were significantly elevated compared with baseline in the suspension laryngoscopy group but not the iLMA group. No significant complications were seen in either group. The authors concluded that the iLMA was a safe alternative to conventional suspension laryngoscopy.

Hashmi and colleagues[47] reported the use of the LMA and fiberoptic laryngoscopy in six patients with history of or physical findings predictive of difficult intubation and found excellent conditions, and were able to manage several patients with limited pulmonary reserve undergoing laser resection of subglottic stenosis without significant arterial desaturation.

The use of the LMA and fiberoptic laryngoscope for managing inaccessible glottic lesions is a useful technique that should be considered whenever difficult intubation is anticipated. It makes little sense to spend an hour performing an awake fiberoptic intubation only to discover that the lesion cannot be accessed through suspension laryngoscopy when a safe alternative can be implemented with equipment readily available in most operating rooms.

Surgical alteration of the glottic configuration is typically performed under local anesthesia with sedation, as is discussed by Atkins and Mirza elsewhere in this issue. Some patients are not candidates for sedation, and the LMA offers a reasonable option for general anesthesia. Carrau and colleagues[48] reported use of the LMA, with visualization provided by a flexible laryngoscope, to perform medialization laryngoplasty in four patients. Grundler and Stacey[49] reported a similar technique for vocal cord medialization in a 25-year-old man who refused local anesthesia. Razzaq and Wooldridge[50] reported 13 cases of type I thyroplasty performed on patients presenting with unilateral adductor paralysis, typically associated with surgical resection of lung cancer. Only one adverse event attributable to the LMA was encountered: a down-folded epiglottis, which was promptly recognized and corrected. Gardner and colleagues[51] reported the use of the LMA and flexible laryngoscope in the treatment of two children (aged 4 and 8 years) requiring vocal cord medialization.

Spiegel and Rodriguez[52] reported 31 cases in which the LMA with fiberoptic laryngoscopy was used during cosmetic chondrolaryngoplasty to avoid inadvertent damage to the anterior commissure. A 22-guage needle was placed through the cartilage to identify the level of the anterior commissure to avoid resection at this level, which would lower the vocal pitch. In one patient, this resulted in a small amount of blood from the puncture site contacting the vocal cords, which triggered immediate laryngospasm. This complication was promptly managed with propofol, 50 mg, and succinylcholine, 20 mg. No patient experienced a change in vocal pitch, and no other complications occurred. The investigators suggested use of topical lidocaine before needle puncture to avoid laryngospasm.

Buckmire and colleagues[53] performed a prospective observational study of clinical improvement after Gore-Tex thyroplasty in 20 patients. Outcomes were assessed with "validated, perceptual, and subjective voice outcome measures," including grade, roughness, breathiness, asthenia, strain of the voice (GRBAS), glottal function index (GFI), and voice-related quality of life (VRQOL). Four patients were judged to be unable to cooperate with sedation and were managed with the LMA with fiberoptic laryngoscopy. These patients underwent temporary injection laryngoplasty and were assessed fiberoptically at their subjective "best post-injection voice" to provide images to guide intraoperative management. In this subgroup, greater improvements were seen in all three indices, although the study lacked statistical power to draw this conclusion. Thus, although intraoperative functional assessment remains the gold standard for laryngeal framework surgery, visual assessment of glottic conformation through the LMA is useful in patients who are unable or unwilling to cooperate with this assessment.

Access to the subglottis and upper trachea in intubated patients is often problematic. Use of high-frequency jet ventilation for tubeless laryngeal surgery is described in another article in this issue. However, this approach is impractical in some patients, and the LMA offers an alternative approach. Maroof and colleagues[54] reported use of the LMA in assessing a laryngeal web in a patient in whom rigid bronchoscopy was abandoned because of concerns about damaging loose teeth. The investigators noted that despite their having no previous experience with the technique, access was easily obtained.

Samet and colleagues[55] reported two cases in which neonates presenting with stridor and retractions were evaluated for tracheomalacia through observation of the subglottis during spontaneous ventilation after placing a 2-mm rigid endoscope through a size 1 LMA. The authors observed the LMA permitted observation of tracheal collapse while administering volatile anesthetics and oxygen, permitting safe management in infants weighing less than 5 kg.

Adelsmayr and colleagues[56] reported resection of a high tracheal stenosis with combined use of the LMA and high frequency jet ventilation via a catheter placed through the LMA. Jameson and colleagues[57] reported use of a GaAlAs laser fiber passed through a bronchoscope placed through an iLMA for ablation of a subglottic mass occluding 50% of the trachea. Brimacombe and Dunbar-Reid[58] noted the resistance to airflow was 2.1-fold higher with appropriately sized ETT than with LMA when a fiberoptic bronchoscope was placed through the device. This issue becomes significant when suction is applied, because the negative pressure to which the lung is exposed is greater when an ETT is used.

The LMA can be seen to offer advantages as a conduit for accessing the glottis when direct laryngoscopy is impossible. It offers the advantage of permitting delivery of oxygen and anesthetics while leaving an unobstructed view of the glottis. Given the frequency with which the LMA is currently used in anesthesia, anesthetists with no familiarity with the device are rare, and comfort with advanced uses of the LMA can be acquired rapidly.

LMA for Thyroidectomy

Injury to the recurrent laryngeal nerve is a known complication of thyroidectomy. Monitoring of vocal cord function can be achieved with special endotracheal tubes with electromyogram electrodes, although these add complexity and expense to the procedure. The first mention of the use of the LMA with fiberoptic observation of vocal cord movement was by Tanigawa and colleagues[59] in a letter to the editors of *Anesthesiology* describing 10 patients who had undergone this technique. Transient laryngospasm was observed in two patients. A month later, Greatorex and Denny,[60] in the first of four papers over a 10-year period from Queen Elizabeth Hospital in Norfolk, United Kingdom, reported 13 consecutive cases managed with the LMA as the initial airway. In one case, an adequate seal could not be obtained, and an ETT was placed. In another, the LMA was displaced on manipulation of a large tumor, and the LMA was replaced with an ETT. In six of the cases, the LMA was used as a conduit for passing a fiberoptic laryngoscope to permit identification of the recurrent laryngeal nerve with the nerve stimulator. In two of these cases, identification of the nerve was only possible using this approach. The investigators commented on the advantages of this technique and the ability to manage thyroidectomy cases with the LMA. Hobbiger and colleagues[61] subsequently published their results in 97 consecutive patients, among whom 7 required ETT. No patients experienced postoperative laryngeal nerve dysfunction.

Palazzo and colleagues[62] described the use of the LMA and fiberoptic laryngoscope to evaluate patients with prolonged tracheal compression for tracheomalacia. In six patients judged at high risk for tracheomalacia, observation of the trachea through the LMA permitted five to be managed without tracheostomy. These patients had no respiratory complications postoperatively. The authors noted that because of the ability to evaluate the trachea, these patients were spared elective tracheostomy. Shah and colleagues[63] reviewed 150 consecutive thyroidectomies performed over the 10-year experience. Of these, six were intubated due to preoperative factors, three were intubated after induction when an adequate seal could not be obtained with the LMA, and two were intubated intraoperatively when displacement of the trachea caused an irretrievable loss of LMA seal (neither of these patients experienced significant desaturation). In 64 of the patients, fiberoptic confirmation of recurrent laryngeal nerve function was performed. No patient experienced postoperative vocal complications.

Hillermann and colleagues[64,65] described a technique using a 5-mm microlaryngeal endotracheal tube with an LMA placed behind it, permitting a greater degree of airway control while allowing visual confirmation of vocal cord function. In a series of 30 patients, the superior and laryngeal nerves were identified in all patients, and only one patient (with active thyroiditis) experienced new onset of nerve palsy. The authors noted that 24% of their patients met exclusion criteria for use of the LMA, but all were managed without intraoperative airway events.

Eltzschig and colleagues[66] reviewed 363 consecutive thyroidectomies performed over an 18-month period by a single surgeon. Of these cases, 36 were excluded for preoperative factors, including tracheomalacia, gastroesophageal reflux disease, and unfamiliarity of the anesthesiologist with the LMA. Of the 327 cases performed with the LMA, 16 experienced respiratory events, only three of which were resolved with tracheal intubation. Vocal cord monitoring was performed in 326 of the cases, and nerve identification was achieved solely by nerve stimulation in 10. The only new-onset nerve palsy occurred in the group in which observation was not performed. The rate of one nerve injury in 363 cases was one of the lowest rates of nerve injury ever reported for thyroid surgery. The investigators noted that if the nerve had been sectioned in the 10 cases in which nerve identification was obtained solely through observing the vocal cords, the rate of nerve injury would have been 3%, which is the typical value seen in thyroid surgery without monitoring. The investigators noted that the technique required no additional equipment or personnel, and the procedures were typically accomplished more quickly because of shorter induction and emergence times. They further noted that maintaining the head in a more neutral position was useful in avoiding laryngeal edema from excessive pressure of the LMA on the glottis, but that with attention to proper LMA placement and avoidance of light anesthesia, the rate of intraoperative respiratory compromise requiring intubation was extremely low.

Scheuller and Ellison[67] reported a series of eight patients in whom 13 fiberoptic identifications of the recurrent laryngeal nerve were performed. In 5 of these, a structure believed to be the nerve was found not to be the functional branch, and the true functional branch was identified on further exploration. Pott and colleagues[68] reported 27 cases of thyroidectomy in which the LMA was used. In a single case, the LMA could not achieve an adequate seal and an ETT was placed. In six cases, stridor was experienced in association with traction on the thyroid; in two of these, the surgical team was requested to release tension to permit ventilation. No adverse outcomes were associated with these events, and the authors recommended attention to laryngeal rotation during traction on the thyroid.

The use of the LMA with fiberoptic evaluation of vocal cord function with nerve stimulation is an economical means of achieving a low rate of vocal cord dysfunction. It may permit evaluation of the airway when tracheomalacia is suspected. In centers that embrace the technique, anesthesiologists must be comfortable with placement of the LMA and be prepared to transition to an ETT if adequate ventilation is not achieved. Surgeons must be willing to accept less neck extension and to limit retraction force when it compromises gas exchange. Provisions must be made for monitoring in patients in whom the LMA cannot be used.

SUMMARY

The use of LMA and its variants in ENT procedures have been extensively described in case reports, retrospective reviews, and randomized clinical trials. Although patients certainly exist for whom the LMA is contraindicated, many will experience better results with the LMA because of the features delineated in this article. Practitioners should acquire initial skill with the device in more routine settings, just as endotracheal intubation is not a skill initially learned in patients who have large glottic lesions, have undergone external beam therapy, or have "kissing tonsils." When used appropriately, none of the practices described in this article should be considered deviations from the standard of care for ENT procedures in the modern era.

REFERENCES

1. Brimacombe J. The advantages of the LMA over the tracheal tube or facemask: a meta-analysis. Can J Anaesth 1995;42:1017–23.
2. Tait AR, Pandit UA, Voepel-Lewis T, et al. Use of the laryngeal mask airway in children with upper respiratory tract infections: a comparison with endotracheal intubation. Anesth Analg 1998;86:706–11.
3. von Ungern-Sternberg BS, Boda K, Schwab C, et al. Laryngeal mask airway is associated with an increased incidence of adverse respiratory events in children with recent upper respiratory tract infections. Anesthesiology 2007;107:714–9.
4. Burgess GE, Cooper JR, Marino RJ, et al. Laryngeal competence after tracheal extubation. Anesthesiology 1979;51:73–7.
5. Tanaka A, Isono S, Ishikawa T, et al. Laryngeal reflex before and after placement of airway interventions: endotracheal tube and laryngeal mask airway. Anesthesiology 2005;102:20–5.

6. Duff BE. Use of the laryngeal mask airway in otologic surgery. Laryngoscope 1999;109:1033–6.

7. Ayala MA, Sanderson A, Marks R, et al. Laryngeal mask airway use in otologic surgery. Otol Neurotol 2009;30:599–601.

8. Daum RE, O'Reilly BJ. The laryngeal mask airway in ENT surgery. J Laryngol Otol 1992;106:28–30.

9. Williams PJ, Thompsett C, Bailey PM. Comparison of the reinforced laryngeal mask airway and tracheal intubation for nasal surgery. Anaesthesia 1995;50:987–9.

10. Webster AC, Morley-Forster PK, Janzen V, et al. Anesthesia for intranasal surgery: a comparison between tracheal intubation and the flexible reinforced laryngeal mask airway. Anesth Analg 1999;88:421–5.

11. Ahmed MZ, Vohra A. The reinforced laryngeal mask airway (RLMA) protects the airway in patients undergoing nasal surgery—an observational study of 200 patients. Can J Anaesth 2002;49:863–6.

12. Kaplan A, Crosby GJ, Bhattacharyya N. Airway protection and the laryngeal mask airway in sinus and nasal surgery. Laryngoscope 2004;114:652–5.

13. Atef A, Fawaz A. Comparison of laryngeal mask with endotracheal tube for anesthesia in endoscopic sinus surgery. Am J Rhinol 2008;22:653–7.

14. Al-Mazrou KA, Abdullah KM, ElGammal MS, et al. Laryngeal mask airway vs. uncuffed endotracheal tube for nasal and paranasal sinus surgery: paediatric airway protection. Eur J Anaesthesiol 2010;27:16–9.

15. Williams PJ, Bailey PM. Comparison of the reinforced laryngeal mask airway and tracheal intubation for adenotonsillectomy. Br J Anaesth 1993;70:30.

16. Webster AC, Morley-Forster PK, Dain S, et al. Anaesthesia for adenotonsillectomy: a comparison between tracheal intubation and the armoured laryngeal mask airway. Can J Anaesth 1993;40:1171–7.

17. Heath ML, Sinnathamby SW. The reinforced laryngeal mask airway for adenotonsillectomy. Br J Anaesth 1994;72:728–9.

18. Williams PJ, Bailey PM. The reinforced laryngeal mask airway for adenotonsillectomy. Br J Anaesth 1994;72:729.

19. Hern JD, Jayaraj SM, Sidhu VS, et al. The laryngeal mask airway in tonsillectomy: the surgeon's perspective. Clin Otolaryngol Allied Sci 1999;24:122–5.

20. Keller C, Brimacombe J. The influence of head and neck position on oropharyngeal leak pressure and cuff position with the flexible and the standard laryngeal mask airway. Anesth Analg 1999;88:913–6.

21. Brimacombe JR, Keller C, Gunkel AR, et al. The influence of the tonsillar gag on efficacy of seal, anatomic position, airway patency, and airway protection with the flexible laryngeal mask airway: a randomized, cross-over study of fresh adult cadavers. Anesth Analg 1999;89:181.

22. Gravningsbråten R, Nicklasson B, Raeder J. Safety of laryngeal mask airway and short-stay practice in office-based adenotonsillectomy. Acta Anaesthesiol Scand 2009;53:218–22.

23. Kretz FJ, Reimann B, Stelzner J, et al. The laryngeal mask in pediatric adenotonsillectomy. A dangerous toy or a medical advance? Der Anaesthesist 2000;49:706–12.

24. Hatcher IS, Stack CG. Postal survey of the anaesthetic techniques used for paediatric tonsillectomy surgery. Paediatr Anaesth 1999;9:311–5.

25. Ecoffey C, Auroy Y, Pequignot F, et al. A French survey of paediatric airway management use in tonsillectomy and appendicectomy. Paediatr Anaesth 2003;13:584–8.

26. Clarke MB, Forster P, Cook TM. Airway management for tonsillectomy: a national survey of UK practice. Br J Anaesth 2007;99:425–8.
27. Allford M, Guruswamy V. A national survey of the anesthetic management of tonsillectomy surgery in children. Paediatr Anaesth 2009;19:145–52.
28. Dexter TJ. The laryngeal mask airway: a method to improve visualisation of the trachea and larynx during fibreoptic assisted percutaneous tracheostomy. Anaesth Intensive Care 1994;22:35–9.
29. Tarpey JJ, Lynch L, Hart S. The use of the laryngeal mask airway to facilitate the insertion of a percutaneous tracheostomy. Intensive Care Med 1994;20:448–9.
30. Lyons BJ, Flynn CG. The laryngeal mask simplifies airway management during percutaneous dilational tracheostomy. Acta Anaesthesiol Scand 1995;39:414–5.
31. Sustić A, Zupan Z, Antoncić I. Ultrasound-guided percutaneous dilatational tracheostomy with laryngeal mask airway control in a morbidly obese patient. J Clin Anesth 2004;16:121–3.
32. Verghese C, Rangasami J, Kapila A, et al. Airway control during percutaneous dilatational tracheostomy: pilot study with the intubating laryngeal mask airway. Br J Anaesth 1998;81:608–9.
33. Dosemeci L, Yilmaz M, Gürpinar F, et al. The use of the laryngeal mask airway as an alternative to the endotracheal tube during percutaneous dilatational tracheostomy. Intensive Care Med 2002;28:63–7.
34. Ambesh SP, Sinha PK, Tripathi M, et al. Laryngeal mask airway vs endotracheal tube to facilitate bedside percutaneous tracheostomy in critically ill patients: a prospective comparative study. J Postgrad Med 2002;48:11–5.
35. Craven RM, Laver SR, Cook TM, et al. Use of the Pro-Seal LMA facilitates percutaneous dilatational tracheostomy. Can J Anaesth 2003;50:718–20.
36. Linstedt U, Möller F, Grote N, et al. Intubating laryngeal mask as a ventilatory device during percutaneous dilatational tracheostomy: a descriptive study. Br J Anaesth 2007;99:912–5.
37. Linstedt U, Zenz M, Krull K, et al. Laryngeal mask airway or endotracheal tube for percutaneous dilatational tracheostomy: a comparison of visibility of intratracheal structures. Anesth Analg 2010;110:1076–82.
38. Higgs A, Clark E, Premraj K. Low-skill fibreoptic intubation: use of the Aintree catheter with the classic LMA. Anaesthesia 2005;60:915–20.
39. Pinar E, Calli C, Oncel S, et al. Preoperative clinical prediction of difficult laryngeal exposure in suspension laryngoscopy. Eur Arch Otorhinolaryngol 2009; 266:699–703.
40. Saravanappa N, Ward VM, Harries ML. Deliberate removal of incisor teeth to allow access for laryngoscopy. J Laryngol Otol 2006;115:302–3.
41. Wareing MJ, Fisher EW, Manning RH, et al. The extraction and re-implantation of teeth for the difficult laryngoscopy. J Laryngol Otol 1994;108:44–5.
42. Brimacombe J, Sher M, Laing D, et al. The laryngeal mask airway: a new technique for fiberoptic guided vocal cord biopsy. J Clin Anesth 1996;8:273–5.
43. Kanagalingam J, Hurley R, Grant HR, et al. A new technique for the management of inaccessible anterior glottic lesions. J Laryngol Otol 2003;117:302–6.
44. Windfuhr JP, Remmert S. Intubation laryngeal mask: atraumatic diagnostic tool in suspension laryngoscopy. Acta Otolaryngol 2005;125:100–7.
45. Chang CH, Kim MK, Nam SB. The use of the LMA Fastrach system as a guidance tool for inaccessible glottic lesion biopsies. Acta Anaesthesiol Scand 2007;51: 1130–1.
46. Chang CH, Bai SJ, Kim MK, et al. The usefulness of the laryngeal mask airway Fastrach for laryngeal surgery. Eur J Anaesthesiol 2010;27:20–3.

Laser Surgery and Fire Hazards in Ear, Nose, and Throat Surgeries

David S. Sheinbein, MD*, Robert G. Loeb, MD

KEYWORDS

- Fire triangle • Airway fires • Laser surgery
- Operating room fires • Fire management/prevention
- Anesthesiology

Fires in the operating room are a potential hazard to patients and operating room personnel. Data published in the *Health Devices* in 2009 estimate that there are approximately 550 to 650 surgical fires occurring in the United States each year.[1] Although this is an extremely small percentage of the total annual surgical cases (approximately 65 million each year), operating room fires can have devastating results. In 2003, the Joint Commission published a sentinel event alert, Preventing Surgical Fires, which prompted increased awareness in the surgical community. The American Society of Anesthesiologists has created a task force on operating room fires, and the American College of Surgeons has included surgical fire prevention as a session at its annual conference.

There are several ways in which an operating room fire can lead to injury. Operating room fires can produce significant thermal injury, leading to partial-thickness or full-thickness burns, the latter requiring skin grafting. Destruction of the skin and mucous membranes predisposes the burnt victim to fluid and electrolyte loss, heat loss, and infection. Swelling and edema of the airway are common after any degree of burn in the airway and can lead to life-threatening airway obstruction. Toxins released from burning plastics can also cause inhalation injuries and/or asphyxiation. These toxins include hydrogen, chloride, cyanide, phenols, aldehydes, and other complex hydrocarbons. In addition, most operating room fires result in incomplete combustion, which produces and releases partially oxidized molecules, such as toxic carbon monoxide, acidic free hydrogen, and unburned carbon or soot.

The fire triangle has become the standard for diagramming the 3 necessary components for combustion (**Fig. 1**). The triangle includes an oxidizer, an ignition source, and

Department of Anesthesiology, University of Arizona College of Medicine, PO Box 245114, Tucson, AZ 85724, USA
* Corresponding author.
E-mail address: sheinbein@gmail.com

Anesthesiology Clin 28 (2010) 485–496
doi:10.1016/j.anclin.2010.07.006   **anesthesiology.theclinics.com**
1932-2275/10/$ – see front matter © 2010 Elsevier Inc. All rights reserved.

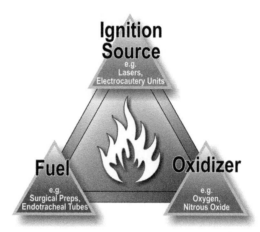

Fig. 1. The "fire triangle" diagramming the 3 necessary components for combustion.

a fuel. When these 3 elements interact under the proper conditions, a fire occurs. These 3 elements are often present in the operating room during surgery. When these elements are in close proximity, there is a high potential of an operating room fire. Anesthesia providers typically supply oxidizers, such as oxygen, nitrous oxide, and air. Surgeons can provide a source of ignition, typically in the form of an electrosurgical unit (ESU), lasers, an electrocautery unit, or a fiberoptic light source. A defibrillator can spark and ignite a fire. Common fuels in the operating room include alcohol-rich prepping agents, surgical drapes and gauzes, tubes and masks, and even gastrointestinal gases and hair.

One of the first steps that the anesthesia staff can do to decrease the risk of operating room fires is to control the oxidizers. Ambient air can support the combustion of many potential fuels in the operating room. Ambient air is composed of 21% oxygen and 78% nitrogen, with fractional percentages of argon, carbon dioxide (CO_2), and other gases. Although air contains enough oxygen to support combustion, oxygen-enriched atmospheres (ie, pure oxygen or air-oxygen mixtures) greatly enhance the rate of ignition and combustion. These oxygen-enriched atmospheres are often created when oxygen concentrations above that in ambient air are provided to patients via routes such as nasal cannulas, face or laryngeal masks, or endotracheal tubes. Oxygen-enriched environments are involved in most operating room fires and present an often-unsuspected fire risk during head, neck, and airway surgeries. Oxygen-enriched atmospheres lower the temperature at which fuels ignite, and cause fires to burn more intensely and spread more quickly. Nitrous oxide also supports combustion by exothermic disassociation, releasing heat and oxygen. Operating room fires involving mixtures of nitrous oxide and oxygen are as easily ignited and as severe as fires involving 100% oxygen. For these reasons, the fire risk when nitrous oxide is mixed with oxygen should be considered equivalent to those risks associated with administering 100% oxygen.

In 2009, the Emergency Care Research Institute (ECRI) along with the Anesthesia Patient Safety Foundation supported the following new guidelines on controlling oxygen delivery during head, face, neck, and upper chest surgery.[1] Use only air for open delivery to the face as long as spontaneously breathing sedated patients can maintain their blood oxygen saturation without extra oxygen. However, if the patient cannot maintain an adequate blood oxygen saturation level without supplemental oxygen, the airway must then be secured with an endotracheal tube or a laryngeal mask airway (LMA). The goal is to prevent an oxygen-enriched environment under the drapes. The traditional practice of openly delivering 100% oxygen to the patient should be discontinued, with limited exceptions. For those cases in which the patient is sedated and spontaneously breathing and open supplemental oxygen is required, the minimal inspired oxygen concentration needed to maintain an adequate blood oxygen saturation level should be used. Ideally, oxygen concentration should be kept at less than 30%. If 100% oxygen must be delivered, it is recommended to lower the oxygen concentration to 30% before using an electrocautery or other potential ignition sources. It might take several minutes to lower the oxygen concentration under the drapes. Delivering 5 to 10 L of supplemental air under the drapes may help wash out extra oxygen. It has also been suggested to scavenge gas from the surgical site with suction and, if possible, to tent the drapes around the patient's head to promote air circulation. Preventing oxygen buildup beneath and within the drapes does more than decrease the chance of fire; it also decreases the intensity of the fire if one starts.[2]

When using a nasal cannula or face mask, an auxiliary flow meter that is only capable of delivering 100% oxygen should not be used. A blended oxygen/air system is recommended to deliver the minimum concentration of oxygen necessary to maintain adequate blood oxygen saturation. A venturi tube has also been suggested for delivering air/oxygen mixtures.[3] During those cases in which open oxygen delivery is mandatory, the ECRI suggests 3 options: (1) use an oxygen-air blender, which is the simplest and most reliable; (2) use a 3-gas anesthesia machine that has a common gas outlet and take the blended gas from the common gas outlet; (3) use the breathing circuit on an anesthesia machine if the machine does not have an available common gas outlet.[1] In the situation using a breathing circuit, a nasal cannula or facemask is attached to the Y-piece of the breathing circuit with a 5-mm endotracheal tube connector. The adjustable pressure-limiting valve is closed completely so that the air/oxygen mixture flows into and pressurizes the breathing circuit, causing flow through the nasal cannula or facemask. The pressure in the breathing circuit (usually below 30 cm H_2O) limits the maximum flow to the patient (approximately 4 L/min through a typical nasal cannula). A standard oxygen analyzer on the inspiratory limb of the anesthesia machine displays the delivered oxygen concentration.[4]

Ignition sources provide the thermal energy that can start a fire. Understanding and controlling ignition sources in the operating room is a key to fire prevention. ESUs are the most common ignition source for fires in the operating room. These units use a high-frequency electric current at the electrode tip to cut or cauterize tissue. It is not just the electrode tip that can ignite a fire; sparking from the electrode cables during a procedure can also cause fire. According to the ECRI, there has never been a report of a fire when using a bipolar ESU, likely secondary to the low power and lack of arcing at the tips of the forceps. To minimize the risk of ignition, the ECRI recommends always placing the electrosurgical forceps in a holster or another location away from the patient when not in active use, because many operating room fires are started by the accidental activation of an ignition source that is temporarily not being used. The ESU should only be activated by the person using it and when the tips are in direct view, and then should be deactivated before leaving the surgical site. Insulating sleeves should never be used over the electrode tips, such as catheters or packing material, because they can cause flame flare-ups. Contaminated electrosurgical active electrodes should be disconnected and removed from the surgical field.

Surgical lasers are cited to be the second most frequent ignition source in operating room fires. The fires caused by surgical lasers are frequently serious, and a deeper

Norton endotracheal tube, the Xomed Laser-Shield endotracheal tube, the Laser-Guard protective wrap, and the Bivona Fome-Cuff endotracheal tube. The Xomed Laser-Shield was involved in at least 3 airway fires, one that resulted in death, before it was withdrawn from the market.[12] Special laser-resistant endotracheal tubes that are still commercially available include the Xomed Laser-Shield II (Medtronic ENT, Jacksonville, FL, USA), the Sheridan Laser-Trach endotracheal tube (Hudson RCI/Teleflex Medical, Research Triangle Park, NC, USA), the Rüsch Lasertubus endotracheal tube (Teleflex Medical, Research Triangle Park, NC, USA), and the Mallinckrodt Laser-Flex endotracheal tube (Covidien-Nellcor, Boulder, CO, USA).

The Norton tube is a reusable completely nonflammable tube that some departments may still have in stock. The tube is constructed of spiral wound stainless steel and has no cuff. The shaft of the Norton tube is not airtight. The pharynx may be packed against the tube to provide a seal for positive pressure ventilation. However, making a good seal can compromise ventilation. Also, the large size and stiffness of the tube may make surgical exposure and laryngoscope positioning difficult.

The Laser-Shield II endotracheal tube is constructed from PVC that is wrapped with protective aluminum foil and a smooth fluoroplastic overwrap. The endotracheal tube is intended for use with CO_2 and KTP lasers and is available in 4-, 4.5-, 5-, 5.5-, 6-, 6.5-, 7-, 7.5-, and 8-mm internal diameter (ID) sizes. The single-cuff system contains methylene blue to indicate cuff perforation. In a laboratory study, the protected area of this endotracheal tube withstood continuous CO_2 laser exposure at 20 W (although the fluoroplastic overwrap did vaporize where it was impacted).[13]

The Laser-Trach endotracheal tube is constructed from red rubber (ie, contains latex) that is embossed with copper foil to diffuse laser energy. The endotracheal tube is intended for use with CO_2 and KTP lasers, is available in 4-, 5-, and 6-mm ID sizes, and has a single-cuff system. This tube is the only laser-resistant endotracheal tube with depth markings. In a laboratory evaluation, this endotracheal tube withstood 40 W of continuous CO_2 laser exposure for 60 seconds; however, it did ignite and burn vigorously when exposed to a high-power Nd:YAG laser beam.[14]

The Lasertubus endotracheal tube is made of soft white rubber (ie, contains latex) that is covered by a protective layer of microcorrugated silver foil and absorbent Merocel sponge (Medtronic, Jacksonville, FL, USA) around the distal 17 cm of the tube. The tube has a dual cuff-within-a-cuff system and is available in 4-, 5-, 6-, 7-, and 8-mm ID sizes. It is intended for use with all types of medical lasers, including CO_2, Nd:YAG, and argon. In a preliminary report by Sosis and colleagues,[15] the protected section of this endotracheal tube withstood 90 seconds of exposure to an Nd:YAG laser set at 25 W and to a CO_2 laser set at 75 W.

The Laser-Flex endotracheal tube has a crimped stainless steel shaft; cuffed versions have 2 PVC cuffs arranged in series. The purpose of having 2 cuffs is that the distal cuff remains intact even if the proximal one is damaged by the laser. The cuffs are inflated by 2 separate pilot lines that run along the inside of the endotracheal tube. This endotracheal tube is intended for use with CO_2 and KTP lasers. Uncuffed tubes are available in 3-, 3.5-, and 4-mm ID sizes; cuffed tubes are available in 4.5-, 5-, 5.5-, and 6-mm ID sizes. Sosis and Heller[16] demonstrated that the shaft of this tube was not affected by a 69-W CO_2 laser beam applied for 1 minute. However, the shaft was compromised by the Nd:YAG laser when operated at high power.

Current recommendations from the ECRI to minimize ignition source risks during laser surgery are as follows. Always limit the laser output to the lowest clinically acceptable power density and pulse duration. Test fire the laser before starting the procedure. The laser should be placed in a standby mode when not in active use and deactivated and placed in a standby mode before removing it from the surgical site. The laser should be activated only by the person using it and only when the tip is in direct view. If possible, use surgical devices designed to minimize laser reflectance and use a laser backstop to reduce the likelihood of tissue injury distal to the surgical site. Never clamp the fibers to the drapes because clamping can break the fibers. When performing laser surgery through an endoscope, pass the laser fiber through the scope and test it before inserting the endoscope into the patient. When performing lower airway surgery, the laser fiber tip should be visible and clear of the end of the bronchoscope or endotracheal tube before using the laser. Even when flammable materials are not used in the path of the laser, it should be recognized that charred tissue and laser plume can ignite in an oxygen-rich environment.[17] For this reason, the oxygen concentration at the point of laser impact should be kept below 40% when possible.

In addition to ESUs and lasers, other common ignition sources in the operating room include electrocautery and fiberoptic light sources. Electrocautery is the use of an electric current to heat a wire or scalpel blade to a high temperature to cauterize or cut tissues and vessels. The tissue is not a part of the electric circuit, and it does not create an electrical arc. Wire electrocautery probes operate at extremely high temperatures, above incandescence, and have been involved in operating room fires. No surgical fires have been reported with blade-style electrocautery. The ECRI recommends the proper disposal of electrocautery materials to prevent operating room fires (ie, break off the cauterizing wire and cap the pencil).

Another potential ignition sources are the argon beam cautery (ABC) device and argon plasma coagulation (APC) device. The APC device is typically used through an endoscope, whereas the ABC device is used during open surgery. Both devices deliver a stream of argon gas that is ionized by a high-voltage discharge. A high-frequency electric current is conducted from the device through the ionized gas (plasma) to coagulate or cauterize the tissue target. There is no contact of the device probe with the surface of the tissue. Although there are no case reports of fires during the use of these devices, a laboratory study confirmed that bronchoscopic APC can ignite airway stents in a high-oxygen environment.[18]

Fiberoptic light sources can also start fires. Incandescent light energy is collected and directed into an optical fiber to illuminate specific areas during surgery. These light sources can produce hundreds of watts of light power and thus have the potential to ignite a fire. It is recommended that active fiberoptic cables never be placed on drapes or other flammable materials. The fiberoptic light source should be placed in a standby mode or the light source should be turned off before disconnecting its cables.

Minimizing and managing fuel sources are imperative to reduce the risk of operating room fires. Common fuel sources in the operating room include prepping agents, linens, dressings, ointments, operating room equipment, and the patient's body tissue and hair. Saline-soaked gauze, cottonoids, or towels can be used to shield flammable material from ignition sources. However, wet material may dry out fairly rapidly and then increase rather than decrease the risk of fire. Prepping agent fires are caused by the ignition of flammable vapors at the surgical site. Pooling, spilling, or wicking of flammable liquid preparations (eg, alcohol and DuraPrep [3M, Maplewood, MN, USA]) should be avoided. Spilled and/or pooled agent should be soaked up and removed from the patient. Towels used to absorb dripped preparation solution should be removed, and adequate time should be allowed for flammable liquid preparations to evaporate and fully dry before draping; this drying process can take up to 5 minutes. For surgery around the head, face, neck, and upper chest, coating the patient's hair with a water-soluble surgical lubricating jelly can make the hair nonflammable.

Oropharyngeal and tracheal surgical procedures are considered high risk for fires because an ignition source may be used in the presence of an oxygen-enriched environment. Fires during tonsillectomy occur when an oxygen-enriched environment is allowed to build up in the oropharynx and potential fuels, such as endotracheal tubes, disposable plastic suction cannulas, and rubber catheters, become ignited usually through a flame flare-up of desiccated tissue or blood on the electrosurgical tip. The risk of fire during tonsillectomy can be reduced by using an oxygen concentration of less than 30% and by preventing a leak around the endotracheal tube with either a cuffed endotracheal tube or spontaneous ventilation through an LMA. If an oxygen concentration greater than 30% is used, the oropharynx should be suctioned with a metal cannula before using the ESU. Some mouth gags used during tonsillectomy are designed to separate and protect the endotracheal tube from the areas where the ESU is going to be used on the tissue. Although these gags protect the tube itself from igniting, sponges should be moistened and kept moist throughout the use of the ESU to render the other materials present less flammable.

Fires during tracheostomy can occur if the electrosurgical or electrocautery instruments are used to enter the oxygen-enriched trachea, which can ignite the endotracheal tube. It is recommended to lower the oxygen concentration to 30% before entering the trachea, if possible, and to use a scalpel or scissors rather than the ESU or electrocautery instruments to make the tracheal incision (**Fig. 2**).

A fire in the operating room requires an immediate and planned response from the operating room personnel. Immediately announcing that there is a fire to the operating room team is crucial. Once the fire has been recognized, stop the flow of all airway gases to the patient. In most fires, removing the oxidizer causes the fire to go out or at least burn less intensely. Next, remove all burning material from the patient and have another team member extinguish them. A CO_2 fire extinguisher can be used if it is readily available. Removal of burning or burnt materials prevents the patient from suffering further burn injuries from the heat of the materials after the fire is put out. The patient must then be cared for quickly. The anesthesia staff should restore breathing, using air initially, until all possible sources of fire are addressed. The surgeon should evaluate the patient and care for his or her injuries. The patient should be evacuated if the room poses a danger to the patient secondary to the smoke or fire damage. Although rare, if the fire is not quickly controlled, notify the operating room front desk and call the fire department. After evacuating the patient, isolate the room by closing the door and shutting off the power and medical gases.

For small fires not on or near the head, face, or neck, remove the burning material and extinguish the fire by patting it out with a towel or gloved hand. If the fire is in the airway, immediately stop the manual or mechanical ventilation to prevent pushing hot gases and/or flames further down the bronchial tree and simultaneously pull out the endotracheal tube and disconnect it from the breathing circuit. Make sure to remove any other material that may have been placed in the airway during surgery. Instruct another operating room team member to extinguish these materials. Next, pour saline or water into the airway to cool the tissues and make certain that the fire is completely extinguished in the airway. Reestablish the airway by resuming ventilation with air initially, making certain nothing is left burning in the airway, and then switching to 100% oxygen. Using oxygen before ensuring that the fire is not completely extinguished could lead to reignition of the fire. Finally, examine the airway, determine the extent of damage, and treat appropriately.

The acronym RACE (Rescue, Alert, Confine, and Evacuate) is helpful in operating room fire management. The patient should be rescued from the fire. Extra help may be needed to disconnect the patient from devices to remove him or her from the

ONLY *YOU* CAN PREVENT SURGICAL FIRES
Surgical Team Communication Is Essential

The applicability of these recommendations must be considered individually for each patient.

At the Start of Each Surgery:

▶ Enriched O_2 and N_2O atmospheres can vastly increase flammability of drapes, plastics, and hair. Be aware of possible O_2 enrichment under the drapes near the surgical site and in the fenestration, especially during head/face/neck/upper-chest surgery.

▶ Do not apply drapes until all flammable preps have fully dried; soak up spilled or pooled agent.

▶ Fiberoptic light sources can start fires: Complete all cable connections before activating the source. Place the source in standby mode when disconnecting cables.

▶ Moisten sponges to make them ignition resistant in oropharyngeal and pulmonary surgery.

During Head, Face, Neck, and Upper-Chest Surgery:

▶ Use only air for open delivery to the face if the patient can maintain a safe blood O_2 saturation without supplemental O_2.

▶ If the patient cannot maintain a safe blood O_2 saturation without extra O_2, secure the airway with a laryngeal mask airway or tracheal tube.

Exceptions: Where patient verbal responses may be required during surgery (e.g., carotid artery surgery, neurosurgery, pacemaker insertion) and where open O_2 delivery is required to keep the patient safe:

— At all times, deliver the minimum O_2 concentration necessary for adequate oxygenation.

— Begin with a 30% delivered O_2 concentration and increase as necessary.

— For unavoidable open O_2 delivery above 30%, deliver 5 to 10 L/min of air under drapes to wash out excess O_2.

— Stop supplemental O_2 at least one minute before and during use of electrosurgery, electrocautery, or laser, if possible. Surgical team communication is essential for this recommendation.

— Use an adherent incise drape, if possible, to help isolate the incision from possible O_2-enriched atmospheres beneath the drapes.

— Keep fenestration towel edges as far from the incision as possible.

— Arrange drapes to minimize O_2 buildup underneath.

— Coat head hair and facial hair (e.g., eyebrows, beard, moustache) within the fenestration with water-soluble surgical lubricating jelly to make it nonflammable.

— For coagulation, use bipolar electrosurgery, not monopolar electrosurgery.

During Oropharyngeal Surgery (e.g., tonsillectomy):

▶ Scavenge deep within the oropharynx with a metal suction cannula to catch leaking O_2 and N_2O.

▶ Moisten gauze or sponges and keep them moist, including those used with uncuffed tracheal tubes.

During Tracheostomy:

▶ Do not use electrosurgery to cut into the trachea.

During Bronchoscopic Surgery:

▶ If the patient requires supplemental O_2, keep the delivered O_2 below 30%. Use inhalation/exhalation gas monitoring (e.g., with an O_2 analyzer) to confirm the proper concentration.

When Using Electrosurgery, Electrocautery, or Laser:

▶ The surgeon should be made aware of open O_2 use. Surgical team discussion about preventive measures before use of electrosurgery, electrocautery, and laser is indicated.

▶ Activate the unit only when the active tip is in view (especially if looking through a microscope or endoscope).

▶ Deactivate the unit before the tip leaves the surgical site.

▶ Place electrosurgical electrodes in a holster or another location off the patient when not in active use (i.e., when not needed within the next few moments).

▶ Place lasers in standby mode when not in active use.

▶ Do not place rubber catheter sleeves over electrosurgical electrodes.

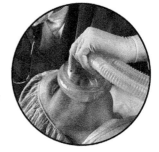

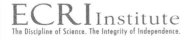 **ECRI**Institute
The Discipline of Science. The Integrity of Independence.

Developed in collaboration with the
Anesthesia Patient Safety Foundation.

Source: New Clinical Guide to Surgical Fire Prevention. *Health Devices* 2009 Oct;38(10):319. ©2009 ECRI Institute
More information on surgical fire prevention, including a downloadable copy of this poster, is available at www.ecri.org/surgical_fires

Fig. 2. Fire prevention recommendations in the operating room. (Reprinted with permission. Copyright © 2009, ECRI Institute. www.ecri.org. 5200 Butler Pike, Plymouth Meeting PA 19462. 610-825-6000.)

EMERGENCY PROCEDURE
EXTINGUISHING A SURGICAL FIRE

Fighting Fires ON the Surgical Patient
Review before every surgical procedure.

In the Event of Fire on the Patient:

1. Stop the flow of all airway gases to the patient.

2. **Immediately remove the burning materials** and have another team member extinguish them. If needed, use a CO_2 fire extinguisher to put out a fire on the patient.

3. Care for the patient:
   —Resume patient ventilation.
   —Control bleeding.
   —Evacuate the patient if the room is dangerous from smoke or fire.
   —Examine the patient for injuries and treat accordingly.

4. If the fire is not quickly controlled:
   —Notify other operating room staff and the fire department that a fire has occurred.
   —Isolate the room to contain smoke and fire.

Save involved materials and devices for later investigation.

Extinguishing Airway Fires
Review before every surgical intubation.

At the First Sign of an Airway or Breathing Circuit Fire, Immediately and Rapidly:

1. **Remove the tracheal tube,** and have another team member extinguish it. Remove cuff-protective devices and any segments of burned tube that may remain smoldering in the airway.

2. Stop the flow of all gases to the airway.

3. Pour saline or water into the airway.

4. Care for the patient:
   —Reestablish the airway, and resume ventilating with air until you are certain that nothing is left burning in the airway, then switch to 100% oxygen.
   —Examine the airway to determine the extent of damage, and treat the patient accordingly.

Save involved materials and devices for later investigation.

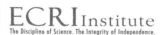

Developed in collaboration with the
Anesthesia Patient Safety Foundation.

Source: New Clinical Guide to Surgical Fire Prevention. *Health Devices* 2009 Oct;38(10):330. ©2009 ECRI Institute
More information on surgical fire prevention, including a downloadable copy of this poster, is available at www.ecri.org/surgical_fires

Fig. 3. Extinguishing a fire in the operating room. (Reprinted with permission. Copyright © 2009, ECRI Institute. www.ecri.org. 5200 Butler Pike, Plymouth Meeting PA 19462. 610-825-6000.)

operating room. Rescuers should not, however, put themselves at risk. Alert all operating room staff of the fire situation and the possible need for evacuation of all patients and personnel from the area. Activate the fire alarm and notify the fire department. Attempt to confine the fire to the operating room in which it occurred by closing all doors and turning off power and shutting off all medical gases to that operating room. Also, evacuate the incident operating room and, if necessary, the entire surgical suite (**Fig. 3**).

Operating room fires are rare but can be devastating. These fires can occur during almost any surgical procedure but are more likely during airway surgery (especially with a laser), during head and neck surgery (especially if supplemental oxygen is administered by nasal cannula or face mask), and if volatile flammable liquids (such as alcohol-based preparation solutions or ether-based barrier dressings) are used. Each team in the operating room (ie, anesthesia, surgery, and nursing) has special expertise and responsibility in preventing and responding to a fire. Fires can be prevented by ongoing education and an interdisciplinary discussion of risks and responsibilities prior to each high-risk case.

REFERENCES

1. S.F.S Initiatives. New clinical guide to surgical fire prevention. Health Devices 2009;38:314–32.
2. Hamza M, Loeb RG. Fire in the operating room. J Clin Monit Comput 2000;16: 317–20.
3. Loeb RG. Supplying sub-100% oxygen gas mixtures during monitored anesthesia care: respiratory monitoring and use of a venturi device. Anesth Analg 2006;103:1048 [author reply: 1048].
4. Lampotang S, Gravenstein N, Paulus DA, et al. Reducing the incidence of surgical fires: supplying nasal cannulae with sub-100% O_2 gas mixtures from anesthesia machines. Anesth Analg 2005;101:1407–12.
5. Mosely H, Oswal V. Laser biophysics. In: Oswal V, Remacle M, editors. Principles and practice of lasers in otorhinolaryngology and head and neck surgery. The Hague (The Netherlands): Kugler; 2003. p. 5–20.
6. Wegrzynowicz ES, Jensen NF, Pearson KS, et al. Airway fire during jet ventilation for laser excision of vocal cord papillomata. Anesthesiology 1992;76:468–9.
7. Santos P, Ayuso A, Luis M, et al. Airway ignition during CO_2 laser laryngeal surgery and high frequency jet ventilation. Eur J Anaesthesiol 2000;17:204–7.
8. Frochaux D, Rajan GP, Biro P. [Laser-resistance of a new jet ventilation catheter (LaserJet) under simulated clinical conditions]. Anaesthesist 2004;53:820–5 [in German].
9. Hunsaker DH. Anesthesia for microlaryngeal surgery: the case for subglottic jet ventilation. Laryngoscope 1994;104:1–30.
10. Sosis MB. Anaesthesia for laser. Int Anesthesiol Clin 1990;28:119–31.
11. Sosis MB, Dillon FX. Saline-filled cuffs help prevent laser-induced polyvinyl chloride endotracheal tube fires. Anesth Analg 1991;72:187–9.
12. Bauman N. Problem laser endotracheal tubes: one company is plagued with lawsuits and accidents. J Clin Laser Med Surg 1990;8:4–7.
13. Green JM, Gonzalez RM, Sonbolian N, et al. The resistance to carbon dioxide laser ignition of a new endotracheal tube: Xomed Laser-Shield II. J Clin Anesth 1992;4:89–92.
14. Sosis MB, Braverman B, Caldarelli DD. Evaluation of a new laser-resistant fabric and copper foil-wrapped endotracheal tube. Laryngoscope 1996;106:842–4.

15. Sosis M, Kelanic S, Caldarelli D. An in vitro evaluation of a new laser resistant endotracheal tube: the Rüsch Lasertubus. Anesthesiology 1997;87S:A483.

16. Sosis MB, Heller S. A comparison of special endotracheal tubes for use with the CO_2 laser. Anesthesiology 1988;69:A251.

17. Juri O, Frochaux D, Rajan GP, et al. [Ignition and burning of biological tissue under simulated CO_2-laser surgery conditions]. Anaesthesist 2006;55:541–6 [in German].

18. Colt HG, Crawford SW. In vitro study of the safety limits of bronchoscopic argon plasma coagulation in the presence of airway stents. Respirology 2006;11:643–7.

Anesthesia for Functional Endoscopic Sinus Surgery: A Review

Martha R. Cordoba Amorocho, MD[a],*,
Anthony Sordillo, DDS, DMD[b]

KEYWORDS

- Functional endoscopic sinus surgery • Anesthesia
- Rhinosinusitis • Chronic sinusitis

Rhinosinusitis is the inflammation of the nose and paranasal sinuses. The paranasal sinuses provide lubrication to the upper respiratory tract, resonance to the voice, and lighten the weight of the skull. The sinuses are maintained in a healthy state by a mucociliary transport mechanism that keeps the protective layer of mucous flowing out of the sinuses through the sinus ostia. When the sinus ostia are blocked, because of allergy, inflammation, infection, irritation, abnormal anatomy, or any other cause of obstruction, infection may ensue.[1]

Sinus surgery has been performed for more than 100 years. Functional endoscopic sinus surgery (FESS) has been practiced only in the last 25 years. It was previously thought that once the mucosa had become chronically inflamed, it was irreversibly damaged and had to be removed. Previous surgical techniques involved radical and extensive removal of the diseased paranasal sinus lining. These procedures left scars and caused significant bruising and discomfort.

Messerklinger[2] showed that the paranasal sinuses drain in a consistent pattern into an area called the ostiomeatal complex. The ostiomeatal complex is composed of the middle meatus under the middle turbinate. All of the paranasal sinuses drain into this region, either directly or in the case of the posterior ethmoid and the sphenoid sinus, indirectly, having ostia situated more posteriorly. The rationale behind FESS is that localized pathology in the ostiomeatal complex blocks the ostia and leads to inflammation in the dependent sinuses. Using fiberoptic endoscopes, it is possible to access

The authors have nothing to disclose.
[a] Department of Anesthesiology and Critical Care, Brigham and Women's Hospital, 75 Francis Street, Boston, MA 02115, USA
[b] Department of Anesthesiology, Massachusetts Eye and Ear Infirmary, 243 Charles Street, Boston, MA 02114, USA
* Corresponding author.
E-mail addresses: martacordoba@gmail.com; mcordoba-amorocho@partners.org

Anesthesiology Clin 28 (2010) 497–504
doi:10.1016/j.anclin.2010.07.007   **anesthesiology.theclinics.com**
1932-2275/10/$ – see front matter © 2010 Elsevier Inc. All rights reserved.

the postnasal space from the anterior nares and to remove the ostiomeatal blockage.[3] FESS restores normal sinus ventilation and mucociliary function in a minimally invasive manner.

FESS has a high rate of success, approximately 90%, for symptomatic improvement in patients with medically refractory chronic rhinosinusitis.[4] The FESS approach is now used for a variety of surgical indications in addition to chronic sinusitis. These indications include resection of inverted papilloma, skull base tumor excision, treatment of vascular malformations associated with hereditary hemorrhagic telangiectasia, and transsphenoidal pituitary tumor resection.

Complications of FESS relate to the proximity of the paranasal sinuses to the orbit and brain. Fortunately, the reported complications are few, at least when the surgery is performed by experienced surgeons. Major complications include cerebrospinal fluid leak, penetration into the brain, intracranial infection, blindness resulting from orbital trauma or damage to the optic nerve, hemorrhage requiring transfusions or surgical control, carotid artery injury, and anosmia. Minor complications include nasolacrimal duct injury, synechiae, subcutaneous emphysema, ostial stenosis or closure, and minor bleeding.[5–7]

LOCAL VERSUS GENERAL ANESTHESIA

When FESS was originally introduced, it was thought that patients should preferably be operated under local/topical anesthesia with combined sedation. In this manner, patients would be able to signal any kind of pain or discomfort, alerting and allowing the surgeon to minimize trauma and complications.[8,9] However, FESS has evolved over time and many of the surgical procedures currently performed under FESS might be prolonged and accompanied by bleeding. The use of CT guidance and the evolution of the surgical technique have allowed surgeons to become much more aggressive with the scope of their endoscopic procedures, including skull base surgery and the resection of areas not easily anesthetized with local anesthesia. Anxiety, stress, and discomfort may ensue in both patients and surgeons. In such cases, an increased risk of complications might occur. For a good surgical result and experience, it is crucial that both patients and surgeons feel comfortable during the operation. Currently, local anesthesia is still considered suitable for minor procedures in selected patients, but general anesthesia is preferred for most cases to meet more challenging surgical needs.[10]

PREOPERATIVE EVALUATION

Preoperative evaluation should be performed in every case in which an anesthesia provider will be involved and should be the same for local and general anesthesia. There are specific areas of concern involved in preoperative evaluation.

- Concern exists when there is a history of obstructive sleep apnea (OSA) and the use of continuous positive airway pressure (CPAP) devices at home, in which case they may be needed during postoperative recovery time. Unfortunately in many cases, CPAP use in the perioperative period is complicated by the surgery itself and discouraged by the surgical team.
- Patients' cardiovascular status and the ability to tolerate locally applied vasoconstrictors is an area of concern, as in patients with a history of coronary artery disease (CAD) or cardiac arrhythmias.
- Concern exists with chronic steroid use, in which case patient management is controversial. Patients undergoing FESS likely do not routinely need a stress

dose of steroids as long as they receive their usual daily maintenance steroid dose, either orally preoperatively or the equivalent intravenous dose intraoperatively.[11]

- Concern exists with the probability of a life-threatening bronchospasm associated with the triad of nonsteroidal antiinflammatory drug (NSAID) sensitivity, asthma, and nasal polyps.

INDUCTION CONSIDERATIONS

Various methods are used to reduce bleeding and to guarantee better visibility during FESS.

If tolerated, it is better to position patients in reverse Trendelenburg, with at least 15° of the head up. In the context of deliberate hypotension, the use of reverse Trendelenburg position has additional risks. Blood pressure will most likely drop even further because this position allows for venous decongestion of the upper part of the body by increasing venous pooling of blood in the lower extremities. Blood pressure measurements obtained at the level of the heart, either with a blood pressure cuff or an arterial line transducer, will not reflect the real and lower values of the most elevated body parts, such as the head.

Preoperative steroid administration in cases of severe nasal polyposis will have antiinflammatory and antiedematous effects, improving the visibility during FESS.[12]

Injected and topical vasoconstrictors are applied to the nasal mucosa to relieve postoperative pain, decrease blood loss and mucosal congestion, and enhance hemostasis. Commonly used vasoconstrictors include cocaine, epinephrine, and phenylephrine. Cocaine has local anesthetic and vasoconstrictor properties. Systemic absorption of cocaine and the vasoconstrictors contained in local anesthetics occurs, so it is important to monitor patients carefully during surgery.[13,14] Vasoconstrictor-related side effects include hypertension, hypotension, tachycardia, bradycardia, and other arrhythmias. Cocaine and other vasoconstrictors should be used with great caution or avoided altogether in patients with a history of CAD, myocardial infarction, congestive heart failure, irregular heart rhythm, poorly controlled hypertension, and in those taking monoamine oxidase inhibitors.

The combined use of topical phenylephrine and beta-blockade in FESS or any other ear, nose, and throat (ENT) surgery deserves special consideration. Aggressive use of topical phenylephrine to decrease blood loss during ENT surgery may produce α-agonist– induced hypertension. If cardiac depressant therapy, such as β-blockers and potentially calcium channel blockers, is used to treat this phenylephrine-induced hypertension, cardiac output may worsen and result in pulmonary edema or other potentially lethal outcomes. It is recommended that the initial dose of phenylephrine should not exceed 0.5 mg in adults (4 drops of a 0.25% solution) or 20.0 mcg/kg in children (up to 25 kg). If severe hypertension is present after administration of phenylephrine, antihypertensive agents that are direct vasodilators or α-antagonists are the appropriate therapy.[15]

Hypotension induced by epinephrine under general anesthesia is seldom mentioned, but temporary marked hypotension is proven to be induced in a predictable manner, lasting no longer than 4 minutes after local infiltration with epinephrine-containing local anesthetics.[16,17] Considering the potential for adverse side effects, the effect of topical application of epinephrine 1:100,000 has been studied and it may actually be able to provide a similar hemostatic effect as intranasal injection during FESS.[18]

AIRWAY: ENDOTRACHEAL TUBE VERSUS LARYNGEAL MASK AIRWAY

An endotracheal tube (ETT) would seem like the first and only option for FESS, considering its seal would protect the airway more effectively than a laryngeal mask airway (LMA); however, this may not be true. Blood can still pass along the outer surface of the ETT to the level of the vocal cords and subglottis. Direct comparisons of lower airway contamination by fiberoptic examination at the end of nasal surgery have shown that patients managed with a flexible LMA, using spontaneous ventilation, are less or at least as likely to have blood in the airway compared with patients managed with an ETT.[19–22]

It seems logical to extrapolate the results of LMA use for nasal surgery into FESS and it has been done with good results.[23] In the end, the choice between an ETT and LMA for FESS depends on the level of comfort and experience of the anesthesiologist and surgeon with each device for this particular surgery; duration of surgery; and patient factors, such as history of obesity, chronic obstructive pulmonary disease, gastroesophageal reflux disease, and previous gastric surgery.

The advantages of using an ETT are its familiarity and ability to secure the airway and provide positive-pressure ventilation if required. The use of an oral RAE tube (Cardinal Health, Dublin, OH, USA) versus a standard ETT allows for less kinking at the mouth. An orally placed RAE or standard ETT positioned in the midline and secured to the chin is often used with a throat pack to reduce blood contamination of the oral airway. At the end of the surgery the pack should be removed and a careful inspection of the oral cavity and postnasal space should be performed. Any clot left behind can be inhaled after removal of the ETT and lead to airway obstruction and even death.[24] Extubation is usually undertaken with patients awake or deep. The advantage of awake extubation for FESS is the return of laryngeal reflexes that allow airway protection from further contamination with blood and secretions. The disadvantage of awake extubation is the possibility of laryngospasm, coughing and bucking with subsequent oxygen desaturation, and increased risk of bleeding. Deep extubation is performed when trying to speed the transfer to the recovery unit and trying to smooth the recovery profile itself. However, deep extubation leaves an unprotected airway and even more, during FESS, the nasal airway is often blocked with surgical packs making it extremely difficult for patients to maintain an airway just dependent on oropharyngeal airflow. If deep extubation is performed, additional suctioning with direct visualization of the glottis, using a regular laryngoscope or even a video laryngoscope, could decrease the risk of aspiration of blood and secretions.

Using a flexible LMA is an advanced use of the device and the anesthesiologist should be familiar with the device before use in FESS. Any incorrect placement, dislodgement during the case, or suboptimal recovery after removal creates the potential for airway obstruction and contamination of the lower airway with blood and secretions. LMA removal is performed once patients are awake and able to open the mouth on command. LMA use for head and neck surgery is reviewed in depth by Mandel in an accompanying article in this issue.

MAINTENANCE OF ANESTHESIA

To reduce the incidence of complications during FESS that may be related to inadequate visualization, it is important to have a surgical field as free of blood as possible. One of the advantages of local anesthesia is reduced mucosal bleeding. Currently, general anesthesia is used more often than local anesthesia because it provides better comfort for patients and optimal operating conditions for surgeons. However, even if the surgery is performed under general anesthesia, local anesthetics are still applied to reduce bleeding.

The use of total intravenous anesthesia (TIVA) with avoidance of inhalational anesthetic reduces bleeding and improves visualization of the surgical field, making TIVA the strongly preferred anesthetic technique for many ENT surgeons. TIVA also has the potential to decrease coughing on emergence and postoperative nausea and vomiting (PONV) in the postoperative period. TIVA may reduce blood loss by maintaining lower blood pressures.[25–27] However, the results of using controlled hypotension during FESS are contradictory, seemingly dependent on the agent used to produce hypotension.

Propofol and remifentanil are safe and improve the quality of the surgical field by reducing blood loss. When inhaled anesthesia using isoflurane and fentanyl was compared with TIVA using propofol and remifentanil, both techniques were equally effective in achieving hypotension, as defined by mean arterial pressures between 60 to 70 mm Hg, but only TIVA was effective in reducing bleeding during FESS.[28] TIVA, with propofol and remifentanil, has also been compared with balanced anesthesia with esmolol during FESS in children, with similar results. Hypotension was sustained at the target of 50 mm Hg in both groups, but intraoperative blood loss and the quality of the surgical field was better in the TIVA group.[29]

Magnesium sulfate has also been shown to produce hypotension effectively and to reduce heart rate, blood loss, and duration of surgery. However, magnesium infusion seems to alter anesthetic dose requirement and to prolong emergence time.[30] On the other hand, sodium nitroprusside does not improve surgical conditions or decrease blood loss when compared with esmolol, even while producing the same degree of hypotension.[31,32]

High frequency jet ventilation (HFJV) is another method to reduce bleeding and to improve visibility during FESS that needs additional investigation. During FESS, HFJV has been achieved using a ventilation cannula inserted through an ETT with a ventilator rate of 150/min, inspiration/expiration ratio of 1:1, and insufflated gas pressure of 2.0 to 2.5 bar (29.4–37.7 psig). When compared with intermittent positive pressure ventilation, HFJV was found to reduce the amount of intraoperative bleeding, maybe as a consequence of increased venous return caused by lower intrathoracic pressures. However, there are concerns regarding HFJV, such as risk of necrotizing tracheobronchitis because of inadequate humidification with high gas flows and cooling of the inspiratory gases at the jet orifice, risk of barotrauma caused by inappropriate airway pressure monitoring or insufficient expiratory airflow, and risk of inadequate ventilation with unpredictable CO_2 levels.[33]

Another technique that has been tried in an attempt to minimize complications during FESS using general anesthesia is the monitoring of intraoperative visual evoked potentials (VEPs). During FESS, injury to the eye and blindness may occur by direct surgical injury or by increased orbital pressure as a result of a retrobulbar hemorrhage. VEPs offer a way of monitoring the function of the visual pathway during surgery and may decrease visual morbidity, including blindness. Current methods to monitor VEPs require placing a lens on the lubricated eye and securing it with Steri-Strips (3M, St Paul, MN, USA). The lens has an attached, small plastic prism and photostimulator. Even when no palpebral stitching is required, the procedure is still cumbersome, requires the use of eye lubricant, precludes the surgeon from accessing the eyes during the surgery, and increases the risks of corneal injury. VEPs are also easily influenced by a variety of anesthetic agents and additional confounding factors other than surgical injury, such as blood pressure, oxygen saturation, and the amount of bleeding. For these reasons, VEPs are not really used in clinical practice.[34]

POSTOPERATIVE CARE

The incidence of postoperative nausea and vomiting after FESS is not well reported. The presence of blood in the stomach, inflammation of the uvula and throat, and the occasional use of opioids for pain control may all be contributing factors. Decompressing the stomach with an orogastric tube before extubation may be helpful in cases with excessive bleeding in which an ETT was used. Other standard treatments for PONV, such as a scopolamine patch, ondansetron, and dexamethasone, should be used depending on patient history and risk factors for PONV.

If a nasal pack is left in place, it is important to remember that patients have a partially or completely obstructed nasal airway, which is particularly significant for patients with OSA who need close observation until complete recovery. Nasopharyngeal airways can be incorporated into the nasal pack to facilitate breathing. In case of severe bleeding, an intravenous cannula should be retained until removal of the nasal pack.

The expected postoperative pain from FESS ranges from mild to moderate, which is related to both surgical trauma and nasal packing. Preoperative local anesthetics are used, but are not enough to alleviate postoperative pain. No differences have been found between infiltration with long acting (bupivacaine) or short acting (lidocaine) local anesthetics.[35,36] The use of nonopioid analgesics after FESS most likely provides similar pain control to opioids.[37] Routine analgesic treatment is usually based on nonopioid analgesics with rescue opioids. Parecoxib administered before discontinuing general anesthesia was not superior to proparacetamol in treating early postoperative pain.[38] Oral acetaminophen and an NSAID/cyclooxygenase 2 inhibitor usually provide safe and effective analgesia. Although this modality of analgesia is agreeable for most of surgeons, a subset may still have concerns regarding increased bleeding risk because of associated pharmacologic platelet dysfunction.

SUMMARY

Functional endoscopic sinus surgery has become one of the most common head and neck procedures performed. Proper anesthetic management is essential for a successful outcome. Different anesthesia techniques are discussed, including local versus general anesthesia, LMA versus ETT, and inhaled anesthesia versus TIVA. The anesthetic plan should be tailored, taking into consideration patient comorbidities, surgeon and anesthesiologist experience, and individual preference. Specific anesthetic goals are to ensure the best possible surgical field and stable cardiovascular and respiratory status during the surgery, upon emergence of anesthesia, and upon recovery.

REFERENCES

1. Archer S. Functional endoscopic sinus surgery. Atlas Oral Maxillofac Surg Clin North Am 2003;11:157–67.
2. Messerklinger W. Background and evolution of endoscopic sinus surgery. Ear Nose Throat J 1994;73:449–50.
3. Slack R, Bates G. Functional endoscopic sinus surgery. Am Fam Physician 1998; 58:707–18.
4. Senior BA, Kennedy DW, Tanabodee J, et al. Long term results of functional endoscopic sinus surgery. Laryngoscope 1998;108:152–7.
5. Cumberworth VL, Sudderick RM, Mackay IS. Major complications of functional endoscopic sinus surgery. Clin Otolaryngol 1994;19:248–53.

6. Sharp HR, Crutchfield L, Rowe-Jones KM, et al. Major complications and consent prior to endoscopic sinus surgery. Clin Otolaryngol 2001;26:33–8.
7. Stammberger H. Results, problems and complications. In: Stammberger H, editor. Functional endoscopic sinus surgery. The Messerklinger technique. Philadelphia: B.C. Decker; 1991. p. 459–77.
8. Lee WC, Kapur TR, Ramsden WN. Local and regional anesthesia for functional endoscopic sinus surgery. Ann Otol Rhinol Laryngol 1997;106:767–9.
9. Fedok FG, Ferraro RE, Kingsley CP, et al. Operative times, postanesthesia recovery times, and complications during sinonasal surgery using general anesthesia and local anesthesia with sedation. Otolaryngol Head Neck Surg 2000; 122:560–6.
10. Gittelman PD, Jacobs JB, Skorina J. Comparison of functional endoscopic sinus surgery under local and general anesthesia. Ann Otol Rhinol Laryngol 1993;102: 289–93.
11. Marik P, Varon J. Requirement of perioperative stress doses of corticosteroids. A systematic review of literature. Arch Surg 2008;143:1222–6.
12. Sieskiewicz A, Olszewska E, Rogowski M, et al. Preoperative corticosteroid oral therapy and intraoperative bleeding during functional endoscopic sinus surgery in patients with severe nasal polyposis: a preliminary investigation. Ann Otol Rhinol Laryngol 2006;115:490–4.
13. John G, Low JM, Tan PE, et al. Plasma catecholamines levels during functional endoscopic sinus surgery. Clin Otolaryngol 1995;20:213–5.
14. Anderhuber W, Walch C, Nemeth E, et al. Plasma Adrenaline concentrations during functional endoscopic sinus surgery. Laryngoscope 1999;109:204–7.
15. Groudine S, Hollinger I, Jones J, et al. New York State Guidelines on the topical use of phenylephrine in the operating room. Anesthesiology 2000;82: 859–64.
16. Yang JJ, Li WY, Wang ZY, et al. Local anesthesia for functional endoscopic sinus surgery employing small volumes of epinephrine-containing solutions of lidocaine produces profound hypotension. Acta Anaesthesiol Scand 2005;49:1471–6.
17. Yang JJ, Wang QP, Wang TY, et al. Marked hypotension induced by adrenaline contained in local anesthetic. Laryngoscope 2005;115:348–52.
18. Lee TJ, Huang CC, Chang PH, et al. Hemostasis during functional endoscopic sinus surgery: the effect of local infiltration with adrenaline. Otolaryngol Head Neck Surg 2009;140:209–14.
19. Ahmed ZM, Vohra A. The reinforced laryngeal mask airway (RLMA) protects the airway in patients undergoing nasal surgery –an observational study of 200 patients. Can J Anaesth 2002;49:863–6.
20. Webster AC, Morley-Foster PK, Janzen V, et al. Anesthesia for Intranasal surgery: a comparison between tracheal intubation and the flexible reinforced laryngeal mask airway. Anesth Analg 1999;88:421–5.
21. Kaplan A, Crosby GJ, Bhattacharyya N. Airway protection and the laryngeal mask airway in sinus and nasal surgery. Laryngoscope 2004;114:652–5.
22. Williams PJ, Thompsett C, Bailey PM. Comparison of the reinforced laryngeal mask airway and tracheal intubation for nasal surgery. Anaesthesia 1995;50: 987–9.
23. Danielsen A, Gravningsbraten R, Olofsson J. Anaesthesia in endoscopic sinus surgery. Eur Arch Otorhinolaryngol 2003;260:481–6.
24. Feldman MA, Patel A. Anesthesia for eye, ear, nose and throat surgery. In: Miller RD, editor. Miller's anesthesia. 7th edition. Philadelphia: Churchill Livingstone; 2010. p. 2357–88.

25. Sivaci R, Yilmaz MD, Balci C, et al. Comparison of propofol and sevoflurane anesthesia by means of blood loss during endoscopic sinus surgery. Saudi Med J 2004;25:1995–8.
26. Eberhart LH, Folz BJ, Wulf H, et al. Intravenous anesthesia provides optimal surgical conditions during microscopic and endoscopic sinus surgery. Laryngoscope 2003;113:1369–73.
27. Blackwell KE, Ross DA, Kapur P, et al. Propofol for maintenance of general anesthesia: a technique to limit blood loss during endoscopic sinus surgery. Am J Otolaryngol 1993;14:262–6.
28. Tirelli G, Bigarini S, Russolo M, et al. Total intravenous anesthesia in endoscopic sinus-nasal surgery. Acta Otorhinolaryngol Ital 2004;24:137–44.
29. Ragab S, Hassanin MZ. Optimizing the surgical field in pediatric functional endoscopic surgery: a new evidence-based approach. Otolaryngol Head Neck Surg 2010;142:48–54.
30. Elsharnouby NM, Elsharnouby MM. Magnesium sulfate as a technique of hypotensive anaesthesia. Br J Anaesth 2006;96:727–31.
31. Jacobi KE, Bohm BE, Rickauer AJ, et al. Moderate controlled hypotension with sodium nitroprusside does not improve surgical conditions or decreased blood loss in endoscopic sinus surgery. J Clin Anesth 2000;12:202–7.
32. Boezaart AP, van der Merwe J, Coetzee A. Comparison of sodium nitroprusside- and esmolol-induced controlled hypotension for functional endoscopic sinus surgery. Can J Anaesth 1995;42:373–6.
33. Gilbey P, Kuyuek Y, Samet A, et al. The quality of the surgical field during functional endoscopic sinus surgery –The effect of the mode of ventilation: a randomized, prospective, double-blind study. Laryngoscope 2009;119:2449–52.
34. Hussain SSM, Laljee HCK, Horrocks JM, et al. Monitoring of intra-operative visual evoked potentials during functional endoscopic sinus surgery (FESS) under general anaesthesia. J Laryngol Otol 1996;110:31–6.
35. Friedman M, Venkatasan TK, Lang D, et al. Bupivacaine for postoperative analgesia following endoscopic sinus surgery. Laryngoscope 1996;106:1382–5.
36. Buchanan MA, Dunn GR, Macdougall GM. A prospective double-blind randomized controlled trial of the effect of topical bupivacaine on post-operative pain in bilateral nasal surgery with bilateral nasal packs inserted. J Laryngol Otol 2005; 119:284–8.
37. Church CA, Stewart C, O-Lee TJ, et al. Rofecoxib versus hydrocodone/acetaminophen for postoperative analgesia in functional endoscopic sinus surgery. Laryngoscope 2006;116:202–6.
38. Leykin Y, Casati A, Rapotec A, et al. Comparison of parecoxib and paracetamol in endoscopic nasal surgery patients. Yonsei Med J 2008;49:383–8.

Anesthesia for Pediatric Airway Surgery: Recommendations and Review from a Pediatric Referral Center

Corey E. Collins, DO[a,b,*]

KEYWORDS

• Pediatric anesthesia • Airway surgery • Tracheostomy
• Laryngotracheal reconstruction • Anesthesia risk
• Spontaneous ventilation anesthesia

The intrinsic risks of surgery on the pediatric airway are significant and well documented. The provider who accepts responsibility for these children should do so with due consideration of the safety of the proposed surgery, the anesthesia department's ability to provide a continuity of care that minimizes risk, and the provision of care within the standards of local medical centers. In this review, the experience of the Massachusetts Eye and Ear Infirmary's Department of Anesthesia is used as a basis for the description of the variety of clinical cases that present to our operating room.

Many clinician readers will recognize the calendar of cases: adenotonsillectomy in obese children with obstructive sleep apnea (OSA); direct laryngoscopy (DL) on the former preterm infant with stridor; foreign body in the airway. Others will have similar experience with tertiary referral cases such as revision laryngotracheal resection or intralaryngeal juvenile recurrent papillomata. For those with low-acuity pediatric practice, the review of perioperative challenges with these examples should serve to illustrate the approach necessary to safely anesthetize these children and contribute to broad competency in the management of the pediatric airway.

[a] Pediatric Anesthesia, Department of Anesthesiology, Massachusetts Eye and Ear Infirmary, 243 Charles Street, Boston, MA 02114, USA
[b] Harvard Medical School, Boston, MA, USA
* Corresponding author. Pediatric Anesthesia, Department of Anesthesiology, Massachusetts Eye and Ear Infirmary, 243 Charles Street, Boston, MA 02114.
E-mail address: corey_collins@meei.harvard.edu

Anesthesiology Clin 28 (2010) 505–517
doi:10.1016/j.anclin.2010.07.008
1932-2275/10/$ – see front matter © 2010 Elsevier Inc. All rights reserved.
anesthesiology.theclinics.com

PEDIATRIC AIRWAY SURGERY INCIDENCE, RISK, AND COMPETENCE

Demographic and incidence data on pediatric airway surgical procedures in the United States are difficult to estimate and would require a survey of each type of surgery considered. The most informative data may be gleaned from analysis of nearly 700,000 tonsillectomies, with or without adenoidectomy, performed in 2006 as the predominate airway surgery in children.[1] Other surgeries are rare by comparison with most complex airway surgeries referred to tertiary centers. The major sources of other data on perioperative adverse events are the American Society of Anesthesiologists (ASA) Closed Claims Database, the Pediatric Perioperative Cardiac Arrest Database, and large single-center outcomes reports (eg, Mayo Clinic), or national registries such as the United Kingdom Report of the National Confidential Enquiry into Perioperative Deaths. Head and neck surgery remains a high-risk arena for pediatric anesthesia, with no significant decline in its representation among ASA closed claims cases across 3 decades.[2] Ostensibly, the higher risk of ear, nose, and throat (ENT) surgery is caused by surgical manipulation of the pediatric airway and the incumbent risk of subsequent airway event. From 1990 to 2000, 23% of damaging events were caused by respiratory events, with 35% of cases associated with ENT surgery. Other datasets do not find this same association with critical events.[3] The British review of perioperative deaths in 1989 clearly advocated for pediatric patients to receive care from experienced, high-volume providers.[4] Clearly, children categorized as high-acuity (ASA 3–5) require significant experience and expertise to minimize risk; a more difficult debate reflects the rare critical event affecting the child who is ASA 1 to 2 having routine ENT surgery.[5,6]

Recognition of risk requires thorough evaluation of each patient and concurrent medical disease. Although preoperative consultation seems to be a requisite step before anesthesia for airway surgery, often children are acutely symptomatic or referred to an airway specialist with extensive disease. In our center, such children are often fast-tracked to the operating room. Concurrent consultations with gastroenterologists and pulmonologists permit rapid evaluation in our aerodigestive disorders clinic; ideally, the child receives a pediatric anesthesia consultation at this time. Thorough evaluation of specific risks for cardiac, neuromuscular, neurologic, or developmental diseases require prompt referral to other specialists. The anesthesia-related risks are often predicted by concurrent disease (**Table 1**).

DIAGNOSTIC PROCEDURES

Frequently, children present with significant respiratory symptoms and require anesthesia to permit a diagnostic procedure. Although most children tolerate flexible nasopharyngoscopy in the ENT clinic, it is less likely that a child will permit an examination below the larynx without general anesthesia or deep sedation.[7] Although diagnostic DL can be completed in minutes, the necessity to ensure safe induction and emergence can add significant time and resources. For example, the child with a history of congenital heart disease may require thorough diagnostic cardiac evaluation despite the brevity of a proposed procedure. Similarly, the clinician is cautioned to minimize instrumentation of the pediatric airway without peripheral intravenous (IV) access to minimize the risk of adverse airway events.

The most common reasons for DL and bronchoscopy are stridor, pulmonary aspiration, dysphagia, dysphonia, croup, recurrent pneumonia, or suspected foreign body aspiration. Younger children are more likely to exhibit stridor, croup, or recurrent choking spells from congenital causes, whereas the older child is more likely to have an acquired condition such as foreign body, pathologic mass, or trauma.

Table 1
Significant preoperative considerations before pediatric airway surgery

Organ System	Comorbid Conditions	Preanesthetic Implications	Intraoperative Adjustments to Consider
Cardiac history	Structural heart disease Cardiac surgery Dysrhythmia history Acute life-threatening events Medications	Assess risks of cardiac arrest, significant dysrhythmia, shunt physiology, paradoxic embolism, response to hypercarbia or hypoxemia	Maintain normocarbia Filter intravenous fluids Consider need for ionotropic support
Pulmonary history	Chronic lung disease Pulmonary hypertension Recent respiratory infection Chronic aspiration	Assess risk of adverse respiratory event	Consider risk/benefit of Fio_2 options Consider effects of spontaneous vs controlled ventilation
Airway history	Difficult ventilation, intubation Syndrome associated with airway difficulty Microstomia, macroglossia, ptossoglossis Retrognathia, temporomandibular joint disease	Assess risk of unexpected difficult mask ventilation or intubation, adverse airway event, desaturation	Prepare for difficult airway Consider surgical airway options Maintain spontaneous ventilation
Neurologic history	Seizure disorder Intracranial pathology	Assess risk of hypercarbia on autoregulation Assess risk of induction techniques	Consider intravenous vs inhalational induction Consider risks of drug interactions Assess seizure risk
Neuromuscular disorders	Hypotonia Mitochondrial myopathies	Assess risks of malignant hyperthermia, sensitivity to anesthetics and analgesics, postoperative respiratory embarrassment	Consider need for clean technique Consider postoperative ventilation Consider increased response to analgesics, neuromuscular blocking drugs
Birth history	Prematurity and associated sequellae	Chronic pulmonary disease, developmental delay, history prolonged intubation	Increases risk of respiratory events, difficult intravenous access
Social issues	Guardianship Behavioral issues Consent Language barriers	Assess resources needed to assist family and child	Need for social-work assistance, interpreters Consider ability of guardian/child to comprehend planned surgery and risks

In our center, triple endoscopies are frequently performed on children of a variety of ages. This includes DL, flexible fiber optic bronchoscopy and esophagogastroduodenoscopy (EGD). Following inhalational induction of anesthesia with sevoflurane and IV cannulation, a DL/rigid bronchoscopy is performed with spontaneous ventilation to assess laryngeal anatomy and function. Specifically, the laryngeal architecture is studied for evidence of laryngeal lesions, clefts, webs, vocal fold movement, and laryngomalacia. Proximal examination of the airway is focused on the subglottis for evidence of stenosis, lesions, and malacia. The examination is terminated with inspection to the carina and proximal bronchi. Spontaneous ventilation yields important information to the surgeon regarding dynamic characteristics of the larynx and airways. Furthermore, the anesthetic can be rapidly decreased to permit vigorous vocal fold movement should vocal cord paralysis be considered. To facilitate longer examinations, it can become necessary to insufflate anesthetic vapor into the hypopharynx via an oral or nasal conduit, or to transition to an IV technique to ensure adequate anesthesia depth. This technique seems preferable to an apneic intermittent intubation technique because it avoids repeated intubation, reduces subsequent mucosal trauma, decreases the risks associated with episodic desaturation, and shortens procedural duration. A total IV technique can provide equivalent conditions, although titration of infusions to such rapidly changing clinical stimulation while avoiding apnea or light anesthesia can be problematic and lead to higher rates of rescue maneuvers such as intubation, interrupted bronchoscopy, or administration of paralytics.

Potential complications during DL/bronchoscopy include laryngospasm, bronchospasm, airway trauma, cardiac dysrhythmia caused by enhanced vagal tone, cardiac events caused by occult or concurrent structural cardiac disease, or aspiration of pulmonary contents. Certainly, adverse airway events are most likely to occur should a light plane of anesthesia occur without careful airway management. Maneuvers that seem to decrease these events include aerosolized lidocaine to the vocal folds and carina to a total dose of less than 3 mg/kg, close observation of the child for any movement or response to the initial stimulation of the airway (placement of tooth guards, insertion of the laryngoscope, engagement of the suspension apparatus), and immediate withdrawal of all equipment with patient response.

Flexible bronchoscopy is next performed via a laryngeal mask airway (LMA) to assess distal airways and obtain bronchial lavage specimens. The LMA serves as a ready conduit for delivery of the bronchoscope to the larynx, permits modest control of respiratory rate and depth through continuous positive airway pressure or assisted ventilation, maintains spontaneous ventilation as needed to document dynamic airway pathophysiology (tracheomalacia), and minimizes additional traumatic irritation to the subglottic airway. The presence of lipid-laden macrophages is suspicious for chronic aspiration of gastric fluid, although the specificity and sensitivity is low. Brushings may be obtained to assess for abnormal mucosal epithelium (eg, cystic fibrosis, Kartagener syndrome). Should an LMA not permit safe bronchoscopy conditions, the study can be performed via an endotracheal tube (ETT), although this may increase resistance to delivery of tidal volumes, limit visualization of the subglottis, or underestimate the degree of tracheomalacia.[8] The diameter of the smallest flexible bronchoscope is 2.5 mm; although this will pass through smaller ETTs (>3.5 mm outer diameter), the procedure is likely to be difficult because of friction, high airway resistance, and increased risk of dislodgement of the ETT. Despite the risks and challenges, an ETT may be preferable in children who are syndromic if the hypopharynx anatomy is abnormal, children with cardiac disease when careful avoidance of hypoxemia and hypercarbia is necessary, a history of difficult mask ventilation or laryngoscopy, or safe ventilation via an LMA is unlikely.

Lastly, an EGD is performed. Airway management is predicated on the child's condition and requirements for a safe procedure, and may include spontaneous ventilation with moderate sedation or general anesthesia. The LMA placed for the fiber optic bronchoscope is often left in situ, the cuff deflated, and the gastroscope passed while the patient breathes spontaneously. Because this procedure is generally performed last in the series, previous adverse events can necessitate a need for more invasive and controlled airway management, especially after instrumentation of the lower airways. For example, vigorous coughing with bronchial lavage may make it unsafe to attempt EGD minutes later. In these cases, an ETT is placed and the anesthetic deepened. Insufflation of the stomach with 10 to 15 cm H_2O air will impede ventilation in a spontaneously breathing child; smaller children or infants often desaturate during this period and may require interventions such as withdrawal of the scope and decompression of the stomach, positive pressure assistance via the LMA, or endotracheal intubation.

Complication rates are low overall for diagnostic procedures and are related to higher ASA classification, younger age, and experience of the anesthesia staff. In our center, these children are routinely discharged the same day.

AIRWAY TRAUMA

Recent advances in public safety initiatives have resulted in significant declines in pediatric trauma resulting from motor vehicle accidents and sports injuries. However, burns and gunshot wounds remain a consistent source of airway injury to children.[9,10] Overall, reports from tertiary pediatric trauma centers suggest that pediatric trauma and subsequent airway surgery is rare. Gwely[11] reported 34 cases of pediatric blunt bronchial trauma between 2000 and 2007. Wootten and colleagues[9] reported 35 patients between 1997 and 2008. In our center, children occasionally present for diagnostic evaluation of airway trauma; more frequently, we are involved in the chronic management of posttraumatic airway reconstruction including laryngotracheal reconstruction, laryngoplasty, excision of suprastomal granulation tissue, or postdecannulation excision of tracheocutaneous fistula. The patients are usually easily managed with age-appropriate induction techniques and airway management dictated by the expected degree of airway stenosis, risk of trauma to scar tissue or granulation tissue, or the risks of positive pressure ventilation versus spontaneous ventilation.

The management of an acute traumatic airway demands careful planning with the surgical and nursing teams. Induction strategy must be discussed, with alternative pathways to a secure airway in place, including immediate surgical airway. Although an awake tracheostomy can be a challenge in a pediatric patient, this may be advisable. Similarly, awake fiber optic examination of the larynx and endotracheal intubation must be considered in certain settings. Numerous sedative strategies may be used to decrease psychological trauma to the child, including small-dose opiate, benzodiazepine, or sedatives such as ketamine (with an antisialagogue), although precise dosing and careful titration is mandatory. Inhalational induction can be considered to protect spontaneous ventilation and support a gentle transition to an anesthetized state.

The risk of a full stomach often confounds clinical decisions; although the morbidity risk for pediatric aspiration with anesthesia induction is low,[12] standard recommendations suggest that rapid sequence induction and intubation remains the gold standard for pediatric airway trauma management.[13] Collective experience with inhaled foreign bodies suggests that inhalational techniques can be safely employed with a full stomach[14] and therefore may be reasonable to consider in a patient with spontaneous ventilation and currently patent airway after trauma. In the setting of a potentially challenging airway and no IV access, our practice is to accept the risk of aspiration of stomach contents and proceed with an inhalational induction, maintain spontaneous ventilation, prepare for immediate surgical airway access, or move immediately to a tracheostomy under mask general anesthesia.

AIRWAY RECONSTRUCTION

Reconstructive surgery for the pediatric patient is necessary following trauma, acquired or congenital stenosis, or failure to maintain a safe airway following endotracheal extubation because of laryngotracheal malacia, webs, or scarring. Excellent reviews on the surgical options are available for the interested clinician.[15–18] Anesthesia management has been reviewed.[19] In our center, the most common indications for airway reconstructions include acquired subglottic stenosis secondary to prolonged endotracheal intubation, severe subglottic tracheomalacia, chronic aspiration of gastric fluid, or prior tracheostomy. Some recent uncommon reasons for laryngeal reconstruction have included a child with junctional epidermolysis bullosa with a scarred occluded larynx, an infant with capillary hemangioma at the cricoid level, and subglottic stenosis resulting from a skateboarding accident in a 12 year old.

In our experience, the anesthetic management begins with a careful preoperative evaluation to assess the cause for airway disease and the risks of possible anesthetic regimens. Specific concerns include cardiac history: structural heart disease and prior cardiac surgery. Communication is critical between team members. Important transition points during surgery must be anticipated. These include (1) tracheal incision and the risk of cough, damage to the endotracheal cuff, or extravasation of air into the mediastinum; (2) risk of pneumothorax or pneumopericardium; (3) replacement of the oral ETT for a proximal ETT with an attendant risk of loss of tracheal lumen; (4) hemorrhage with injury to a thymic, innominate, or thyroid vessel; (5) mainstem bronchus intubation if the ETT is too deeply placed; (6) ETT plugging with blood or mucus, or ETT kinking with high resistance to inspiratory ventilation; and (7) replacement of an oral or nasal ETT with additional risk of trauma to the surgical anastamosis or loss of the airway. Paralysis is often necessary to reduce these risks. At times, flexible fiber optic bronchoscopy is necessary to assist in the diagnosis of acute changes in oxygenation during any of these critical transitions.

Postoperative communication is critical to the safety of the child. Although the surgical team will likely report specific instructions to the intensive care team, the anesthesiologist is wise to discuss airway issues with the intensive care unit (ICU) team as well. Specifically, ease of mask ventilation; laryngoscopic view on initial intubation; recommended LMA size; ETT depth; patient response to intraoperative medications such as opiates; and intraoperative challenges such as desaturation, dysrhythmias, high peak inspiratory pressures, or peripheral venous access should be transmitted. Clear communication regarding such important observations and data improves the safety of the child's recovery and assessment of postoperative abnormalities.

JUVENILE-ONSET RECURRENT RESPIRATORY PAPILLOMATOSIS

Juvenile-onset recurrent respiratory papillomatosis is a rare cause of pediatric airway obstruction and disease; estimated incidence is 4.3 per 100,000 children. Surgical management was reviewed in 2008 by Derkay and Wiatrak.[20] Diagnosis may occur at any age, although 75% of cases are diagnosed by age 5 years, and it is heralded by hoarseness, stridor, or abnormal cry. Lesions rarely threaten the airway initially, although aggressive disease can cause near-complete occlusion of the larynx, spread to the bronchial or pulmonary airways, and undergo malignant transformation to squamous cell carcinoma.[21]

For the child with aggressive disease, frequent anesthetics are needed for debulking procedures, sometimes as often as every 2 to 4 weeks. This frequent surgical requirement is difficult for many children and the anesthesia team must be attentive to the child's needs. Although premedication may be warranted or requested, it is our practice to eschew preoperative sedative administration to optimize postoperative transition through to discharge.

Anesthesia and airway management for patients with respiratory papillomatosis has been described using jet ventilation,[22,23] intermittent apnea/intubation, or tubeless spontaneous ventilation.[24] No technique has been clearly demonstrated as superior, and benefits to each can be argued.

Jet ventilation has been described using a variety of technical innovations to permit the delivery of high-flow, high-pressure gases to the airway using catheters or specifically designed jet laryngoscopes. This technique relies on the delivered gas jet to entrain ambient room gases to supplement the delivery of a tidal volume to the lungs and prevent hypoxia. A recent risk analysis suggests that jet ventilation techniques resulted in less hypoxia than spontaneous ventilation during airway foreign body removal from children less than 5 years of age.[25] This technique is well described as an effective, safe, and advantageous method of ventilating children of all ages during challenging anesthetics.[26,27] However, in a single-center analysis of 661 children and adults undergoing microlaryngoscopy with a variety of anesthetic techniques, Jaquet and colleagues[28] associated jet ventilation with significant barotrauma and the highest rate of laryngospasm. Transtracheal catheters were clearly more problematic than transglottic catheters, likely because of expiratory obstruction.

Intermittent apnea/intubation techniques provide an unobstructed surgical field for laser ablation or electrodissection. The airway is episodically protected with an ETT and oxygenation is normalized between episodes of deoxygenation. Paralytics are typically used, although not required, to establish apnea. This technique exposes the child to an intermittent threat of significant deoxygenation, hypercarbia, and the trauma of repeated subglottic intubation. Some authorities have expressed concern that passing an ETT through mucosa with papillomata can translocate virus to naive distal mucosa and increase the likelihood for more significant subglottic disease. Surgical experience with tracheostomies[29] and airway reconstructions[17] suggests that spread to lower airways is likely a factor of aggressive disease or other intrinsic variables and not surgical intervention of the cervical airway. However, the significant morbidity of papillomata once present in the lower airway argues against routine endotracheal intubation through a diseased glottis.

In our center, we prefer to use spontaneous ventilation techniques for juvenile-onset recurrent respiratory papillomatosis surgery.[30] Anesthesia induction is via gentle inhalation with transition to an IV infusion of propofol and an ultra–short-acting opiate such as remifentanil. Doses are titrated to effect with careful avoidance of apnea. Our typical dosage range is propofol 150 to 250 µg/kg/min with remifentanil 0.05 to 0.1 µg/kg/min. A recent report by Malherbe and colleagues[31] reported higher dose ranges (propofol 200–500 µg/kg/min and remifentanil 0.1–0.2 µg/kg/min). Topical lidocaine (0.5–1 mL 1%–4%) aerosolized spray on the vocal folds and subglottis can minimize sensitivity to manipulation.[32] We use 1% for infants, 2% for smaller children, and 4% in children more than 25 kg to minimize risk of toxicity (>3 mg/kg). As described by Barker and colleagues,[33] a respiratory rate of 10 breaths per minute or less predicts higher risk of subsequent apnea. This study is also useful for predicting the complexity of dosing remifentanil infusion in children of different ages. Even at our center, there are broad dosing ranges among anesthesiologists for these drugs, and all may provide suitable surgical conditions; this underscores the inherent challenge to controlling the response of pediatric patients to anesthetics, predicting the patient response to airway manipulation and surgery, and the role experience plays in the ultimate techniques used for these procedures.

During suspension laryngoscopy and ablative surgery, medications are titrated to effect. Supplemental oxygen can be supplied via the side port of the Lindholm laryngoscope or directly insufflated into the hypopharynx via an ETT in the oral cavity or affixed to a nasal airway. It has been noted by this author that the standard sampling line for end-tidal carbon dioxide monitors can directly attach to the Luer fitting on the Lindholm sideport to permit nonquantitative measurement of end-tidal carbon dioxide and direct monitoring of the respiratory rate. With due attention to pollution of the operating room atmosphere, additional anesthetic depth can be rapidly provided by the insufflation of sevoflurane with the airway gases; this can minimize the inherent delay of IV infusion pharmocodynamics in the setting of sudden changes in surgical stimulation. For example, the complex calculations needed to predict the infusion rates for target-controlled infusion techniques quantify the time inherently necessary to establish steady-state kinetics; once there is a clinical change in stimulation during a procedure, steady state is disrupted and further time is necessary to adjust the systems to reestablish clinical steady-state pharmacology.[34] Using inhalational agents as an adjunct permits nearly immediate end-organ delivery of additional anesthetic and maintains safe and adequate anesthesia depth until infusions can be adjusted. Dosing the agent in this fashion requires some experimentation because no end-tidal measurement can be tracked and clinical response and indicators of anesthetic depth must be relied on.

As with many challenging techniques, vigilance is necessary to decrease complications; a precordial stethoscope and a monitoring hand on the child's abdomen provides important instantaneous and immediate information and feedback regarding the patient's condition throughout the anesthetic course. Clear communication should signs of inadequate anesthesia become apparent permit adjustment in anesthetic depth and likely decrease the apnea rate and expedite surgery. Our surgeons often place a vocal fold spreader to abduct the vocal folds; this device improves visualization and surgical access to more diseased mucosa, although it also increases laryngeal stimulation. Release of this device can precipitate laryngospasm.

After surgery, most children remain spontaneously breathing as they are transferred to the recovery suite. With a young child with aggressive disease, an ETT is occasionally required during emergence. Pain management is often accomplished with topical lidocaine and low-dose morphine (0.05–0.1 mg/kg IV). Ketorolac is an option to avoid narcosis. Nebulized epinephrine can mitigate stridor. Should stridor persist, airway edema, hemorrhage, aspiration, or gastric reflux should be considered and may require helium-oxygen therapy, continuous positive airway pressure ventilation, or endotracheal intubation.

ADENOTONSILLECTOMY

The frequency of adenotonsillectomy in the United States has declined recently, although it remains the most common pediatric surgery.[1] Indications for surgery include recurrent streptococcal pharyngitis/tonsillitis, significant sleep-disordered breathing/OSA with enlarged palatine tonsils, asymmetric tonsillar hyperplasia, or significant enlargement affecting swallowing and speech.[35]

There are a variety of surgical techniques, instruments, interventions, and approaches to the pediatric patient needing tonsillectomy, including unique surgical devices purported to decreasing pain and bleeding,[36] LMA airway management intended to facilitate shorter recovery times and decreased anesthetic requirements,[37] departmental guidelines intended to decrease interoperator variability and adhere to an empiric approach to anesthetic-related decisions,[38] or expert recommendations on the complexities of sleep-disordered breathing and pediatric anesthesia care.[39]

The best anesthetic technique is the culmination of a variety of dependent and independent variables that coexist around a specific patient at a specific time and are incorporated into an anesthetic (and surgical) plan that acknowledges the pertinent identifiable risks and seeks to usher the child through a successful surgical experience with the least realization of possible adverse events. Every provider must accept the responsibility for this process and adjust their care to the limitations of their training, experience, available clinical data, and the environment present at the time of induction.

Preoperative evaluation and data collection have been discussed recently by Lerman.[39] Although these recommendations apply specifically to patients with OSA, the discussion regarding occult cardiac manifestations, the tendency for airway challenges (more difficult mask ventilation, lower Cormack-Lehane airway laryngoscopy score), and the laboratory assays recommended are worth considering in all children having tonsillectomy. Invasive cardiac examination, electrocardiogram, or liver enzyme assay may be reserved for symptomatic, syndromic, or children with a higher pretest probability for an abnormal result.

The general approach to adenotonsillectomy is broadly defined in the available literature; a wide variety of techniques have been studied and compared, underscoring the paucity of objective conclusions. Variations in technique across the world illustrate the many methods of induction (mask, IV, premedication), airway management (ETT, LMA), pain management (opioid based, opioid sparing, local anesthetic based, nonsteroidal antiinflammatory drug), emergence strategy (awake vs deep extubation, no-touch emergence with ETT or LMA), or observation policy (routine day case discharge vs, 23-hour observation vs ICU admission). The debate regarding nonsteroidal antiinflammatory agents is evidence of the substantial barriers to increased uniformity in how we care for patients having tonsillectomy.[40,41]

However, tonsillectomy has incumbent risks for serious perioperative events including aspiration pneumonitis, refractory laryngospasm, exsanguinating hemorrhage, anoxic injury, or death. Survey data from Germany in 2008 shed some light on the characteristics of lethal posttonsillectomy hemorrhages (PTHs), with specific recognition emphasis to treat recurrent bleeding with the highest concern.[42] New York closed claims data confirm that anesthesiologists are more likely to be sued than surgeons after tonsillectomy complications.[43] Postoperative nausea and vomiting occurs in 50% to 89% of these patients because of swallowed blood, opioid administration, or pharyngeal stimulation, and significantly increases the risk of overnight admission, delayed oral intake, and patient satisfaction.[44] With increasing production pressure on operating room teams, these routine cases may receive less preoperative consideration or evaluation, and subtle clues that may predict complications may be missed or dismissed. In addition, constrained staffing models may render resources unavailable to assist should an event occur.

At our center, most children older than 3 years are tracked for same-day discharge by modified Aldrete score readiness criteria. Many children referred to our center exhibit moderate to severe OSA prompting a review of our risk for morphine-related complications. Data from Brown and colleagues[45] provided important awareness of opioid sensitivity among these patients. Most children receive modest morphine and acetaminophen doses for analgesia, dexamethasone and ondansatron for anti-emetic prophylaxis, and deep extubation of the trachea to minimize coughing and airway stimulation when prudent. A small subset of children is observed in the intensive care ward if there are sufficient age, comorbidity, or perioperative concerns.

Our surgeons use all modern surgical options including Coblation, Cold steel, snare, harmonic scalpel, and hot knife.[46] Surgical literature on the various techniques suggests certain benefits to each: Coblation should yield lower pain scores at the risk of slightly higher bleeding rates,[47,48] electrocautery/dissection proponents argue lower bleeding rates but with increased pain scores and duration of analgesic requirement,[49] and harmonic scalpel seems to decrease intraoperative blood loss with comparable pain and recovery scores to other techniques.[36,50] The anesthesia team should be aware of the techniques used in their own centers because some techniques significantly affect operative times, intraoperative blood losses, postoperative pain scores, or time to resumption of oral intake.

Overall, the approach to the patient needing tonsillectomy requires a comprehensive awareness of multiple, sometimes conflicting, concerns, and challenges the anesthesia provider to balance risk with reality. As the science and evidence develops to guide our decisions, improvements will emerge, yielding continued advances in pain management, postoperative nausea and vomiting prophylaxis, decreased adverse event rates, and increased patient satisfaction.

PTH

PTH warrants specific discussion because it is the most common emergency pediatric airway surgery. PTH rates are between 0.5% and 7.5% and are most common in patients more than 15 years of age, boys, patients with frequent infectious tonsillitis, and after hot (electrocautery) versus cold (scalpel) techniques.[51–53] Considering the possibility for lethal hemorrhage,[42] anesthetic management is often required on an emergency basis, with minimal opportunity to evaluate a child's previous anesthetic history or to modify anesthesia-related risks. At a minimum, a rapid sequence induction should be planned with consideration for possible transfusion should uncontrolled bleeding ensue. Care with laryngoscopy is necessary to prevent traumatic dislodgement of an in situ clot. Gastric decompression is performed to assess for occult blood loss and decrease the risk of subsequent pulmonary aspiration. Intravascular fluid repletion is guided by estimated blood loss or vital signs. Other intraoperative concerns include hypovolemic shock, dysrhythmia, or coagulopathy. Occasional vascular abnormalities can precipitate PTH, and proximal vascular control may be needed. After control of the hemorrhage, postoperative nausea can be minimized with irrigation of the oropharynx and the stomach can be suctioned or lavaged. Emergence and extubation of the trachea should occur after return of protective laryngeal reflexes.

Despite the concern for vigorous hemorrhage, the need for transfusion seems to be low following PTH in developed nations. In a retrospective review of ambulatory tonsillectomy in the United States, Bhattacharyya[53] noted that no transfusions were needed after more than 500,000 tonsillectomies, although, in Sweden, a 4-year retrospective review noted that only 3 of 2813 patients required transfusions.[52] However, Windfuhr and colleagues[42] remind us that recurrent bleeding is an ominous sign, and evidence of serious compensated or uncompensated shock requires aggressive resuscitation.

SUMMARY

This article discusses the management of the child having airway surgery, with specific detail on our practice environment at a tertiary specialty pediatric referral center. In our center, the close communication between all teams ensures efficient, safe, and gratifying interventions for our patients. Although many specific technical obstacles arise during the course of any airway procedure, the prepared clinical team can use reasonable tools, experience, and available assistance to choose a safe anesthetic plan. Excellent available references elaborate on the myriad of factors pertaining to any given surgery; however, the higher-order issues included here are intended to expound on these technical issues. The approaches discussed here are not comprehensive or intended to be prescriptive, and in many ways represent the best of our anecdotal wisdom. The reader is offered these items for consideration and scrutiny, criticism and challenge, as the realities of complex patient care continue slowly toward empirical data and conclusive science.

REFERENCES

1. Cullen KA, Hall MJ, Golosinskiy A. Ambulatory surgery in the United States, 2006. Natl Health Stat Report 2009;28(11):1–25.
2. Jimenez N, Posner KL, Cheney FW, et al. An update on pediatric anesthesia liability: a closed claims analysis. Anesth Analg 2007;104(1):147–53.
3. Gobbo Braz L, Braz JR, Modolo NS, et al. Perioperative cardiac arrest and its mortality in children. A 9-year survey in a Brazilian tertiary teaching hospital. Paediatr Anaesth 2006;16(8):860–6.
4. Campling EA, Devlin HB, Lunn JN. The Report of the National Confidential Enquiry into Perioperative Deaths 1989. London: Her Majesty's Stationary Office; 1989.
5. Clark RM. Subspecialty certification in advanced pediatric anesthesiology. ASA Newsletter 2008;72(5):17–9.
6. Pediatric anesthesia practice recommendations. Task Force on Pediatric Anesthesia of the ASA Committee on Pediatric Anesthesia. American Society of Anesthesiologists; 2002. Available at: http://www.asahq.org/clinical/PediatricAnesthesia. pdf. Accessed August 2, 2010.
7. Berkenbosch JW, Graff GR, Stark JM, et al. Use of a remifentanil-propofol mixture for pediatric flexible fiberoptic bronchoscopy sedation. Paediatr Anaesth 2004; 14(11):941–6.
8. Haver KE. Flexible bronchoscopy. In: Haver KE, Brigger MT, Hardy SC, et al, editors. Pediatric aerodigestive disorders. San Diego (CA): Plural Publishing; 2009. p. 16.
9. Wootten CT, Bromwich MA, Myer CM 3rd. Trends in blunt laryngotracheal trauma in children. Int J Pediatr Otorhinolaryngol 2009;73(8):1071–5.
10. Gold SM, Gerber ME, Shott SR, et al. Blunt laryngotracheal trauma in children. Arch Otolaryngol Head Neck Surg 1997;123(1):83–7.
11. Gwely NN. Pediatric traumatic bronchial rupture; results of early and late presentation. Interact Cardiovasc Thorac Surg 2009. [Epub ahead of print].
12. Flick RP, Schears GJ, Warner MA. Aspiration in pediatric anesthesia: is there a higher incidence compared with adults? Curr Opin Anaesthesiol 2002;15(3): 323–7.
13. Langeron O, Birenbaum A, Amour J. Airway management in trauma. Minerva Anestesiol 2009;75(5):307–11.
14. Zur KB, Litman RS. Pediatric airway foreign body retrieval: surgical and anesthetic perspectives. Paediatr Anaesth 2009;19(Suppl 1):109–17.
15. Lando T, April MM, Ward RF. Minimally invasive techniques in laryngotracheal reconstruction. Otolaryngol Clin North Am 2008;41(5):935–46, ix.

16. Cotton RT, O'Connor DM. Paediatric laryngotracheal reconstruction: 20 years' experience. Acta Otorhinolaryngol Belg 1995;49(4):367–72.

17. Boston M, Rutter M, Myer CM 3rd, et al. Airway reconstruction in children with recurrent respiratory papillomatosis. Int J Pediatr Otorhinolaryngol 2006;70(6):1097–101.

18. Santos D, Mitchell R. The history of pediatric airway reconstruction. Laryngoscope 2010;120(4):815–20.

19. Rowe RW, Betts J, Free E. Perioperative management for laryngotracheal reconstruction. Anesth Analg 1991;73(4):483–6.

20. Derkay CS, Wiatrak B. Recurrent respiratory papillomatosis: a review. Laryngoscope 2008;118(7):1236–47.

21. Pransky S, Kang D. Tumors of the larynx, trachea, and bronchi. In: Bluestone C, Stool S, Alper C, editors. Pediatric otolaryngology, vol. 2. 4th edition. Philadelphia: Saunders; 2003. p. 1558–63.

22. Scamman FL, McCabe BF. Supraglottic jet ventilation for laser surgery of the larynx in children. Ann Otol Rhinol Laryngol 1986;95(2 Pt 1):142–5.

23. Patel A, Rubin JS. The difficult airway: the use of subglottic jet ventilation for laryngeal surgery. Logoped Phoniatr Vocol 2008;33(1):22–4.

24. Stern Y, McCall JE, Willging JP, et al. Spontaneous respiration anesthesia for respiratory papillomatosis. Ann Otol Rhinol Laryngol 2000;109(1):72–6.

25. Chen LH, Zhang X, Li SQ, et al. The risk factors for hypoxemia in children younger than 5 years old undergoing rigid bronchoscopy for foreign body removal. Anesth Analg 2009;109(4):1079–84.

26. Mausser G, Friedrich G, Schwarz G. Airway management and anesthesia in neonates, infants and children during endolaryngotracheal surgery. Paediatr Anaesth 2007;17(10):942–7.

27. Rezaie-Majd A, Bigenzahn W, Denk DM, et al. Superimposed high-frequency jet ventilation (SHFJV) for endoscopic laryngotracheal surgery in more than 1500 patients. Br J Anaesth 2006;96(5):650–9.

28. Jaquet Y, Monnier P, Van Melle G, et al. Complications of different ventilation strategies in endoscopic laryngeal surgery: a 10-year review. Anesthesiology 2006;104(1):52–9.

29. Shapiro AM, Rimell FL, Shoemaker D, et al. Tracheotomy in children with juvenile-onset recurrent respiratory papillomatosis: the Children's Hospital of Pittsburgh experience. Ann Otol Rhinol Laryngol 1996;105(1):1–5.

30. Brigger MT, Hartnick CJ. Juvenile onset recurrent respiratory papillomatosis. In: Haver KE, Brigger MT, Hardy SC, et al, editors. Pediatric aerodigestive disorders. San Diego (CA): Plural; 2009. p. 345–52.

31. Malherbe S, Whyte S, Singh P, et al. Total intravenous anesthesia and spontaneous respiration for airway endoscopy in children - a prospective evaluation. Paediatr Anaesth 2010;20(5):434–8.

32. Fahy C. Topical airway anaesthesia for paediatric bronchoscopy. Paediatr Anaesth 2003;13(9):844–5.

33. Barker N, Lim J, Amari E, et al. Relationship between age and spontaneous ventilation during intravenous anesthesia in children. Pediatric Anesthesia 2007;17(10):948–55.

34. Bressan N, Moreira AP, Amorim P, et al. Target controlled infusion algorithms for anesthesia: theory vs practical implementation. Conf Proc IEEE Eng Med Biol Soc 2009;2009:6234–7.

35. Paradise JL. Tonsillectomy and adenoidectomy. In: Bluestone CD, Stool SE, Alper CM, editors. Pediatric otolaryngology, vol. 2. 4th edition. Philadelphia: Saunders; 2003. p. 1210–22.

36. Roth JA, Pincock T, Sacks R, et al. Harmonic scalpel tonsillectomy versus monopolar diathermy tonsillectomy: a prospective study. Ear Nose Throat J 2008;87(6): 346–9.

37. Gravningsbraten R, Nicklasson B, Raeder J. Safety of laryngeal mask airway and short-stay practice in office-based adenotonsillectomy. Acta Anaesthesiol Scand 2009;53(2):218–22.

38. Ewah BN, Robb PJ, Raw M. Postoperative pain, nausea and vomiting following paediatric day-case tonsillectomy. Anaesthesia 2006;61(2):116–22.

39. Lerman J. A disquisition on sleep-disordered breathing in children. Paediatr Anaesth 2009;19(Suppl 1):100–8.

40. Cardwell M, Siviter G, Smith A. Non-steroidal anti-inflammatory drugs and perioperative bleeding in paediatric tonsillectomy. Cochrane Database Syst Rev 2005; 2:CD003591.

41. Allford M, Guruswamy V. A national survey of the anesthetic management of tonsillectomy surgery in children. Paediatr Anaesth 2009;19(2):145–52.

42. Windfuhr JP, Schloendorff G, Baburi D, et al. Lethal outcome of post-tonsillectomy hemorrhage. Eur Arch Otorhinolaryngol 2008;265(12):1527–34.

43. Morris LG, Lieberman SM, Reitzen SD, et al. Characteristics and outcomes of malpractice claims after tonsillectomy. Otolaryngol Head Neck Surg 2008; 138(3):315–20.

44. Edler AA, Mariano ER, Golianu B, et al. An analysis of factors influencing postanesthesia recovery after pediatric ambulatory tonsillectomy and adenoidectomy. Anesth Analg 2007;104(4):784–9.

45. Brown KA, Laferriere A, Moss IR. Recurrent hypoxemia in young children with obstructive sleep apnea is associated with reduced opioid requirement for analgesia. Anesthesiology 2004;100(4):806–10 [discussion: 805A].

46. Cunningham CJ. Tonsillectomy and tonsillotomy: treating the common obstructor. In: Haver KE, Brigger MT, Hardy SC, et al, editors. Pediatric aerodigestive disorders. San Diego (CA): Plural; 2009. p. 141–64.

47. Di Rienzo Businco L, Coen Tirelli G. Paediatric tonsillectomy: radiofrequency-based plasma dissection compared to cold dissection with sutures. Acta Otorhinolaryngol Ital 2008;28(2):67–72.

48. Burton MJ, Doree C. Coblation versus other surgical techniques for tonsillectomy. Cochrane Database Syst Rev 2007;3:CD004619.

49. Glade RS, Pearson SE, Zalzal GH, et al. Coblation adenotonsillectomy: an improvement over electrocautery technique? Otolaryngol Head Neck Surg 2006;134(5):852–5.

50. Kamal SA, Basu S, Kapoor L, et al. Harmonic scalpel tonsillectomy: a prospective study. Eur Arch Otorhinolaryngol 2006;263(5):449–54.

51. Lowe D, van der Meulen J, Cromwell D, et al. Key messages from the National Prospective Tonsillectomy Audit. Laryngoscope 2007;117(4):717–24.

52. Attner P, Haraldsson PO, Hemlin C, et al. A 4-year consecutive study of post-tonsillectomy haemorrhage. ORL J Otorhinolaryngol Relat Spec 2009;71(5): 273–8.

53. Bhattacharyya N. Ambulatory pediatric otolaryngologic procedures in the United States: characteristics and perioperative safety. Laryngoscope 2010;120(4): 821–5.

Review of Anesthesia for Middle Ear Surgery

Sharon Liang, BSc, MBBS[a], Michael G. Irwin, MB, ChB, MD, FRCA[b],*

KEYWORDS
- Anesthesia for middle ear surgery • Controlled hypotension
- Postoperative nausea and vomiting

The middle ear refers to an air-filled space between the tympanic membrane and the oval window. It is connected to the nasopharynx by the eustachian tube and is in close proximity to the temporal lobe, cerebellum, jugular bulb, and the labyrinth of the inner ear. The middle ear contains three ossicles—the malleus, incus and stapes—which are responsible for transmission of sound vibration from the eardrum to the cochlea. This air-filled cavity is traversed by the facial nerve before it exits the skull via the stylomastoid foramen.[1,2] The facial nerve provides motor innervation to the muscles of facial expression.

COMMON MIDDLE EAR SURGERIES

Middle ear disease affects patients of all ages. Common middle ear pathologic conditions requiring surgery in adults include tympanoplasty (reconstructive surgery for the tympanic membrane, or eardrum), stapedectomy or ossiculoplasty for otosclerosis, mastoidectomy for removal of infected air cells within the mastoid bone, and removal of cholesteoma.[2] Common middle ear surgery in children includes tympanoplasty, mastoidectomy, myringotomy, grommet insertion. and cochlear implantation.[2] Some of these procedures can be performed under local anesthesia, although obviously, all surgery can be performed under general anesthesia if necessitated by patient or surgical factors (**Box 1**).

ANESTHETIC CONSIDERATIONS IN MIDDLE EAR SURGERY

Given the unique location, size, and delicate content of the middle ear, great care must be taken during the perioperative period. Special considerations include: provision of a bloodless surgical field, attention to patient's head positioning, airway management,

[a] Department of Anaesthesiology, Queen Mary Hospital, Main Block, Room 43, 2/F, 102 Pokfulam Road, Hong Kong
[b] Department of Anaesthesiology, University of Hong Kong, K424, Queen Mary Hospital, Pokfulam Road, Hong Kong
* Corresponding author.
E-mail address: mgirwin@hku.hk

Anesthesiology Clin 28 (2010) 519–528
doi:10.1016/j.anclin.2010.07.009
1932-2275/10/$ – see front matter © 2010 Elsevier Inc. All rights reserved.

Box 1
Common procedures in middle ear surgery

Local anesthesia

Surgical factors

- Insertion of grommet
- Myringoplasty
- Tympanoplasty
- Stapedotomy
- Stapedectomy
- Ossiculoplasty (IOFNM)
- Mastoidectomy (IOFNM)
- Cholesteoma surgery via intact ear canal (IOFNM)

Patient factors

- Adult
- Patient must be able to understand, cooperate, hear and communicate

General anesthesia

Surgical factors

- Cochlear implantation
- Long operations
- Complicated surgery (eg, extensive scar tissue in middle ear)

Patient factors

- Children
- Mentally unstable, uncooperative patients
- Patients who request general anesthesia

Abbreviation: IOFNM, intraoperative facial nerve monitoring.

---

facial nerve monitoring, the effect of nitrous oxide on the middle ear, a smooth and calm recovery, and prevention of postoperative nausea and vomiting (PONV).[2–5]

A bloodless surgical field is ideal, as even small amounts of blood will obscure the surgeon's view in microsurgery. A combination of physical and pharmacologic techniques is used to minimize bleeding. Attention to patient's head positioning is important to avoid venous obstruction and congestion. In addition, extreme hyperextension or torsion can cause injury to the brachial plexus and the cervical spine.[4] In patients with carotid atherosclerosis, carotid blood flow may be compromised or plaque emboli dislodged, and it is worth auscultating for carotid bruit before surgery. During general anesthesia, the airway can be maintained with a laryngeal mask airway (LMA) or endotracheal intubation; intubation may be more appropriate if extreme neck extension or rotation is required. LMA, however, is a suitable alternative for most middle ear surgery, and a wide range of devices are now available. A well-documented potential complication of otologic surgery is facial nerve paralysis, and a nerve stimulator is often employed for intraoperative monitoring of evoked facial nerve electromyographic activity to aid preservation of the facial nerve. Muscle relaxants should be avoided in this circumstance or, if neuromuscular block is needed to facilitate smooth intubation, choose a dose and an agent (eg, mivacurium no longer manufactured in the United States) that ensures the return of function before the need for neuromuscular monitoring arises.[3–5] It also should be borne in mind that sudden unexpected patient movement may jeopardize the success of surgery, and depth of anesthesia monitoring may be useful. The use of nitrous oxide in middle ear surgery is controversial. A smooth recovery without coughing or straining is important, especially in patients who have undergone reconstructive middle ear surgery to prevent prosthesis displacement. PONV is a common problem after middle ear surgery that can be minimized by appropriate choice of anesthetic technique and antiemetic prophylaxis.[3–5] Most middle ear procedures can be performed as outpatient surgery; thus rapid recovery, good analgesia, and avoidance of nausea and vomiting are essential.[6]

PREOPERATIVE ASSESSMENT

For adults, simple middle ear surgery can be performed under local or general anesthesia, although complicated or long procedures should be performed under general anesthesia. Patients who are able to understand the procedure, and to communicate and cooperate throughout the procedure, are suitable candidates for local anesthesia with or for foregoing sedation.[7] Patients undergoing middle ear surgery often suffer from extensive hearing loss, thus hindering their ability to cooperate, and in this situation, surgery might be better performed under general anesthesia. Leaving the hearing aid in situ in the nonsurgical ear before induction and replacement before emergence may help to minimize anxiety and ease communication. Oral anxiolysis premedication with benzodiazepines can be considered or standard sedation regimens used intraoperatively. A history of cardiovascular disease, hypovolemia, and anemia will limit the degree of hypotension possible. In pediatric patients, in addition to the usual components of preoperative assessment, it is important to check for coexisting syndromes and recent upper respiratory tract infection.[6]

CHOICE OF ANESTHESIA

Four nerves provide innervation to the ear. The auriculotemporal nerve supplies the outer auditory meatus; the great auricular nerve supplies the medial and lower aspect of the auricle and part of the external auditory meatus. The auricular branch of the vagus nerve supplies the concha and the external auditory meatus, and the tympanic nerves supply the tympanic cavity.[1,4]

General or local anesthesia has advantages and disadvantages. Uncomplicated middle ear surgery can be performed under local anesthesia. In a study on local anesthesia in middle ear surgery by Caner and colleagues,[8] patients were premedicated with meperidine and atropine intramuscularly 30 minutes before being taken to surgery, and 5 mg to 10 mg diazepam was given intravenously if the patient was still agitated in the operating room. Two percent lidocaine with 1:10,000 epinephrine was used for infiltration and auriculotemporal/auricular nerve blocks. Seventy-three of the 100 patients said they would prefer local anesthesia for a similar operation in the future. In a similar survey, Yung[7] found the most common discomforts reported were noise during surgery and anxiety, followed by dizziness, backache, claustrophobia, and earache. Despite these discomforts, however, 89% of patients said they would prefer local anesthesia for similar operations in the future. Pain was felt mainly at the beginning of surgery when multiple injections of local anesthetic were given, and perhaps the preoperative application of lidocaine and prilocaine (EMLA) could have assisted in this. For the surgeons, the main advantage of performing middle ear surgery under local anesthesia is the ability to test hearing during surgery, and they also report less bleeding. The main concerns of not performing middle ear surgery under local anesthesia are that patients may not tolerate the discomfort and the possibility of sudden movement. Another drawback is potential toxicity, as near-toxic plasma levels of local anesthetic have been reported in the first 5 minutes following infiltration for tympanoplasty.[9] The head may be obscured by drapes during surgery, and extra vigilance is required for possible respiratory depression or airway obstruction. Supplementary oxygen can be provided with nasal cannulae, and it is also possible to use capnometry or a precordial stethoscope to monitor breathing. Clear plastic drapes may reduce feelings of claustrophobia, and a forced air device can be used to provide some room air ventilation.

Thus, with careful patient selection, adequate preoperative explanation, and appropriate use of sedation, middle ear surgery can be successfully performed under local anesthesia, with high patient and operator satisfaction and acceptance. Benedik and Manohin[10] compared safety and efficacy of propofol versus midazolam for conscious sedation in middle ear surgery. The study demonstrated that propofol was associated with significantly shorter recovery time and better patient and surgeon satisfaction compared with midazolam. Adverse effects of propofol and midazolam, such as respiratory depression, hypotension, and sudden intraoperative movements, are obvious drawbacks.

Alpha-2 agonists such as clonidine or, more recently, dexmedetomidine, may have some advantages, as they produce arousable sedation, analgesia, and a modest reduction in heart rate and blood pressure without respiratory depression, particularly important when the head is obscured by surgical drapes.[11] Dexmedetomidine has been used successfully as the primary sedative with supplementary low-dose propofol and midazolam for monitored anesthesia care during awake thyroplasty, a procedure that requires the patient to verbalize when asked and otherwise remain immobile.[12] Surgeons reported satisfactory operating conditions, and patients had no recall of the procedure and no pain.[12] It also has a role in awake craniotomy.[13] Thus, dexmedetomidine could be used in a similar way for middle ear surgery but has not been widely reported in the literature.

In summary, the advantages of performing middle ear surgery under local anesthesia and conscious sedation include less bleeding, reduced pain in the immediate postoperative period, early mobilization, cost-effectiveness, and the ability to test hearing restoration during surgery.[8]

Despite these advantages, however, and the special concerns of general anesthesia for middle ear surgery outlined earlier, most middle ear surgery is still performed under general anesthesia.

Total intravenous anesthesia (TIVA) versus volatile-based anesthesia for middle ear surgery long has been a subject of debate. Mukherjee and colleagues[14] compared PONV, pain, and conditions for surgery in patients who had undergone middle ear surgery under TIVA using remifentanil and propofol, with technique using fentanyl, propofol, and isoflurane maintenance. More patients in the inhalation group suffered from PONV (25%) versus the TIVA group (8%) in the recovery room. In the early postoperative period, the TIVA group reported higher pain scores and required more morphine in the recovery room, but there was no significant difference at 2, 4, 6, 8, 12, and 18 hours. Conditions for surgery in the TIVA group were reported to be superior. In another study comparing propofol-based anesthesia with inhalation anesthetic techniques in terms of recovery profile and incidence of PONV for middle ear surgery, TIVA was associated with more rapid emergence and less nausea and vomiting.[15,16]

The use of nitrous oxide in anesthetic practice has declined in recent years as a result of concerns over both physical and metabolic effect.[17,18] The use of nitrous oxide in middle ear surgery is particularly controversial. Nitrous oxide is more soluble than nitrogen in blood and in high concentrations enters the middle ear cavity more rapidly than nitrogen leaves, causing a raise in middle ear pressure if the eustachian tube is obstructed.[4,5] During tympanoplasty, the middle ear is open to the atmosphere; thus there is no build-up of pressure, but once a tympanic membrane graft is placed the continued use of nitrous oxide might cause displacement of graft. At the end of surgery, when it is discontinued, nitrous oxide is rapidly absorbed, which may then result in negative pressure also possibly resulting in graft dislodgement, serous otitis media, disarticulation of the stapes, or impaired hearing.[4,5] Thus, the use of nitrous oxide is not recommended in tympanoplasty. Furthermore, a well known adverse effect of nitrous oxide is PONV, and consequently, its use in middle ear surgery may further increase the incidence of PONV above that already associated with this type surgery.

Endotracheal intubation and laryngoscopy during general anesthesia is associated with many potential complications such as sore throat, cough, dental injury, difficult emergence, and use of muscle relaxants for tube insertion.[19] In comparison, the LMA is free from such complications, and a smooth recovery can be attained easily. It also offers advantages of intravenous sedation with less risk of over sedation and obstructive apnea.[20] Safety and efficacy of the LMA were compared with endotracheal intubation in patients who underwent otologic surgery in a retrospective chart review study conducted at a military tertiary care teaching hospital. No major airway complication was reported in either group; a significant decrease in the use of neuromuscular blockers was noted in the LMA group, and total anesthetic time was also shorter in this group. There was no difference in the incidence of PONV or duration of postanesthesia care unit stay.[21] The use of the LMA for head and neck procedures is reviewed in the article by Mandel elsewhere in this issue for further exploration of this topic.

A bloodless operative field is essential, because even a few drops of blood can obscure the surgical field. Physical and pharmacologic techniques are used: a head-up tilt 15° to 20°, avoidance of venous obstruction, normocapnia, and controlled hypotension. Controlled hypotension is defined as a reduction of systolic blood pressure to 80 mm Hg90 mmHg, a reduction of mean arterial pressure to 50 mm Hg to 65 mm Hg in patients without hypertension, or a reduction of 30% of baseline mean arterial pressure in patients with hypertension.[22] A slightly elevated position of the head reduces arterial and venous pressures in areas above the heart; however, it increases the risk of air embolism. In the presence of hypotension, elevating the head will further compromise perfusion of the head and neck region. Pharmacologic agents used for controlled hypotension in ear, nose, and throat surgery include: inhalation anesthetics (eg, isoflurane and sevoflurane), vasodilators (eg, sodium nitroprusside and nitroglycerin), beta adrenoceptor antagonists (labetalol and esmolol), alpha-2 adrenergic agonists (clonidine and dexmedetomidine), opioids (remifentanil),[23] and more recently magnesium sulfate.[24] However, controlled hypotension is not without risk; in addition to the adverse effects of certain pharmacologic agents, it can cause tissue hypoxia by reducing microcirculatory autoregulation of vital organs.

In moderate concentrations, isoflurane lowers blood pressure via a vasodilating effect while preserving cerebral autoregulation. However, at higher concentrations, it causes an increase in intracranial pressure due to increased cerebral blood flow and impairment of cerebral autoregulation.[23] Sevoflurane produces its hypotensive effect by direct vasodilatation without modifying cochlear blood flow.[25,26] In addition, it has a low blood gas solubility and low airway irritability, making it a good agent for gas induction in pediatric patient, although its use is commonly associated with emergence agitation and negative postoperative behavioral changes in this group.[27] In high concentrations, inhalation anesthetics interfere with the measurement of evoked potentials use for facial nerve monitoring.

The vasodilators sodium nitroprusside and nitroglycerin have become less popular because of adverse effects and the availability of better agents. Sodium nitroprusside is very potent and has a fast onset and offset, but it has several serious adverse effects including tachyphylaxis, rebound hypertension, organ ischemia, and cyanide toxicity.[23] Sodium nitroprusside employed as an adjunct to sevoflurane anesthesia in children improved surgical field visibility but provoked lactic acidosis and increased hypercapnia.[23] Nitroglycerin is a short acting nonspecific direct vasodilator of venous and arterial vessels, which does not produce toxic metabolites. Compared with sodium nitroprusside, nitroglycerin is less effective in inducing hypotension and does so more slowly.[23] Both agents require close blood pressure monitoring, preferably with an arterial line.

Labetalol is a competitive antagonist at beta and alpha receptors with a ratio of 7:1. Beta adrenoceptor blockade decreases myocardial contractility and heart rate, while alpha blockade produces vasodilatation.[23] Adverse effects include bronchospasm, prolonged hypotension, and conduction blockade. Esmolol is a short-acting beta-1 adrenoceptor antagonist, which has an onset time of about 3 minutes and duration of action of approximately 10 minutes. It decreases blood pressure by lowering heart rate and reducing renin activity and catecholamine levels.[28] Compared with sodium nitroprusside, beta adrenoceptor antagonists lower blood pressure and reduce blood flow to the middle ear and improve surgical field without metabolic complications.[22]

The alpha-2 adrenoceptor agonists, clonidine and dexmedetomidine, have been discussed earlier in relation to their sedative and analgesic properties. They also markedly reduce catecholamine secretion, are anesthetic sparing, and produce moderate bradycardia and hypotension.[27,29,30] A randomized study investigating the effectiveness of dexmedetomidine in reducing bleeding during septoplasty and tympanoplasty operations demonstrated dexmedetomidine significantly reduced bleeding and fentanyl requirement in septoplasty and reduced fentanyl requirement in tympanoplasty operations, but the decrease in bleeding was not significant.[30] Durmus and colleagues[31] used dexmedetomidine to improve the quality of surgical field in both tympanoplasty and septoplasty, and concluded that dexmedetomidine is a useful adjuvant to decrease bleeding.

Remifentanil is an ultrashort-acting mu receptor agonist. It is able to decrease systemic blood pressure, reduce blood flow to the middle ear, and produce better visibility in the operative field without impairing autoregulation of the middle ear microcirculation.[23,32] The proposed mechanism of action is via central sympathetic blockade. Degoute and colleagues[32] reported that remifentanil combined with sevoflurane in children enabled controlled hypotension, reduced middle ear blood flow, and provided a good surgical field for middle ear surgery with no additional need for other hypotensive agents. Furthermore, remifentanil reduced sevoflurane requirement and helped avoid the use of muscle relaxants. There is some evidence that intraoperative infusion of high doses of remifentanil can cause postoperative hyperalgesia, increasing the postoperative analgesic requirement but this is controversial.[33,34]

Magnesium sulfate is a noncompetitive N-methyl-D-aspartate (NMDA) receptor antagonist with antinociceptive effects, and it inhibits entry of calcium ions into cells. Magnesium sulfate is used as a vasodilator for controlled hypotension. Ryu and colleagues[24] compared remifentanil and magnesium sulfate for middle ear surgery in terms of hemodynamic effects and postoperative pain when combined with sevoflurane. They reported no significant difference over time in mean arterial pressure or heart rate between the drugs. Patients in the magnesium sulfate group had a lower sevoflurane requirement than those receiving remifentanil. Overall, magnesium sulfate was associated with more stable perioperative hemodynamics and produced better analgesia and less PONV compared with remifentanil.

Otologic surgical procedures are associated with facial nerve paralysis, and thus facial nerve protection is an important consideration. Preservation of the facial nerve can be easily confirmed if the patient is not paralyzed,[4] but use of muscle relaxants compromises the interpretation of evoked facial electromyographic activity. Since any sudden movement could jeopardize surgery, it has been suggested that partial neuromuscular blockade as determined by train-of-four peripheral nerve stimulation be used.[35]

Middle ear surgery is associated with a high incidence of PONV. In the absence of antiemetic treatment, 62% to 80% of patients will be afflicted.[36] The etiology of PONV is multifactorial and depends on various factors, including patient demographics, history of PONV, anesthetic technique, use of nitrous oxide, duration of anesthesia and operation, and even surgical experience.[37–39] TIVA reduces PONV compared with using volatile agents.[14] Use of nitrous oxide is associated with a higher incidence of PONV. Patients operated on by residents required more aggressive prophylaxis for PONV than those operated on by specialists.[39] Prophylactic administration of antiemetic medication also decreases the incidence of PONV. Usmani and colleagues[37] compared the efficacy of ondansetron (0.1 mg/kg), dexamethasone (0.15 mg/kg) and a combination of ondansetron (0.1 mg/kg) and dexamethasone (0.15 mg/kg) for prevention of PONV in a randomized double-blind study involving 90 American Society of Anesthesiologists (ASA) I and II patients. They concluded that prophylactic therapy with ondansetron together with dexamethasone is superior to either drug alone. Another study comparing the efficacy of combining granisetron and dexamethasone to either drug alone yielded similar results.[40] This also holds true in pediatric patients.[41,42] Thus, the combination of a selective 5-hydroxy tryptamine type 3 receptor antagonist together with dexamethasone is more effective in preventing PONV than either drug alone. Yeo and colleagues[43] compared the antiemetic efficacy of dexamethasone combined with midazolam and concluded that the addition of midazolam did not significantly reduce the overall incidence of PONV compared with dexamethasone alone. However, the addition of midazolam did lower the incidence of vomiting and the need for rescue antiemetic.[43]

Patients who underwent middle ear surgery under local anesthesia experienced less immediate postoperative pain than those under general anesthesia. A multimodal analgesic approach combining opioids, nonsteroidal anti-inflammatory drugs/COX-2 selective inhibitors, and acetaminophen is generally appropriate. A recent study found blockade of the auricular branch of the vagus nerve with 0.2 mL of 0.25% bupivacaine to be more effective than intranasal fentanyl (2 µg/kg) in management of postoperative pain in infants and children undergoing myringotomy and tube placement.[44]

In conclusion, with careful patient selection, local anesthesia with sedation is a good alternative to general anesthesia for simple middle ear surgery. General anesthesia with TIVA provides a better recovery profile and less nausea and vomiting compared with inhalational anesthesia, and nitrous oxide should be avoided. Remifentanil is a good drug for controlled hypotension and for avoidance of muscle relaxants. If required, partial neuromuscular blockade can still allow facial nerve monitoring during surgery. Combination PONV prophylaxis is more effective than single drug treatment.

REFERENCES

1. Moore KL, Dalley AF. Clinically orientated anatomy. 4th edition. Philadelphia: Lippinocott Williams and Wilkins; 1999.
2. Dhillon RS, Eas CA. Ear, nose, throat, and head and neck surgery: an illustrated colored text. 2nd edition. Edinburgh (UK): Churchill Livingstone; 1999.
3. Deacock AR. Aspects of anaesthesia for middle ear surgery and blood loss during stapedectomy. Proc R Soc Med 1971;64(12):1226–8.
4. Miller RD. Miller's anesthesia, vol. 2. 6th edition. Hershey (PA): Elsevier Churchill Livingstone; 2005.
5. Morgan EG, Mikhail MS, Murray MJ. Clinical anesthesiology. 4th edition. New York: Lange Medical Books/McGraw-Hill; 2006.
6. Bailey CR. Management of outpatient ear, nose and throat surgery. Curr Opin Anaesthesiol 2001;14(6):617–21.
7. Yung MW. Local anaesthesia in middle ear surgery: survey of patients and surgeons. Clin Otolaryngol Allied Sci 1996;21(5):404–8.
8. Caner G, Olgun L, Gultekin G, et al. Local anesthesia for middle ear surgery. Otolaryngol Head Neck Surg 2005;133(2):295–7.
9. Bachmann B, Biscoping J, Adams HA, et al. Plasma concentrations of lidocaine and prilocaine following infiltration anesthesia in otorhinolaryngologic surgery. Laryngol Rhinol Otol (Stuttg) 1988;67(7):335–9.
10. Benedik J, Manohin A. Sedation for middle ear surgery: prospective clinical trail comparing propofol and midazolam. Cent Eur J Med 2008;3(4):487–93.
11. Yuen VM. Dexmedetomidine: perioperative applications in children. Paediatr Anaesth 2010;20(3):256–64.
12. Busick T, Kussman M, Scheidt T, et al. Preliminary experience with dexmedetomidine for monitored anesthesia care during ENT surgical procedures. Am J Ther 2008;15(6):520–7.
13. Poon CC, Irwin MG. Anaesthesia for deep brain stimulation and in patients with implanted neurostimulator devices. Br J Anaesth 2009;103(2):152–65.
14. Mukherjee K, Seavell C, Rawlings E, et al. A comparison of total intravenous with balanced anaesthesia for middle ear surgery: effects on postoperative nausea and vomiting, pain, and conditions of surgery. Anaesthesia 2003; 58(2):176–80.
15. Jellish WS, Leonetti JP, Murdoch JR, et al. Propofol-based anesthesia as compared with standard anesthetic techniques for middle ear surgery. J Clin Anesth 1995;7(4):292–6.
16. Jellish WS, Leonetti JP, Fahey K, et al. Comparison of 3 different anesthetic techniques on 24-hour recovery after otologic surgical procedures. Otolaryngol Head Neck Surg 1999;120(3):406–11.
17. Irwin MG, Trinh T, Yao CL. Occupational exposure to anaesthetic gases: a role for TIVA. Expert Opin Drug Saf 2009;8(4):473–83.
18. Sanders RD, Weimann J, Maze M. Biologic effects of nitrous oxide: a mechanistic and toxicologic review. Anesthesiology 2008;109(4):707–22.
19. Taheri A, Hajimohamadi F, Soltanghoraee H, et al. Complications of using laryngeal mask airway during anaesthesia in patients undergoing major ear surgery. Acta Otorhinolaryngol Ital 2009;29(3):151–5.
20. Duff BE. Use of the laryngeal mask airway in otologic surgery. Laryngoscope 1999;109:1033–6.
21. Ayala MA, Sanderson A, Marks R, et al. Laryngeal mask airway use in otologic surgery. Otol Neurotol 2009;30(5):599–601.

22. Degoute CS, Ray MJ, Manchon M, et al. Remifentanil and controlled hypotension; comparison with nitroprusside or esmolol during tympanoplasty. Can J Anaesth 2001;48(1):20–7.

23. Degoute CS. Controlled hypotension: a guide to drug choice. Drugs 2007;67(7): 1053–76.

24. Ryu JH, Sohn IS, Do SH. Controlled hypotension for middle ear surgery: a comparison between remifentanil and magnesium sulphate. Br J Anaesth 2009;103(4):490–5.

25. Albera R, Ferrero V, Canale A, et al. Cochlear blood flow modifications induced by anaesthetic drugs in middle ear surgery: comparison between sevoflurane and propofol. Acta Otolaryngol 2003;123(7):812–6.

26. Kuratani N, Oi Y. Greater incidence of emergence agitation in children after sevoflurane anesthesia as compared with halothane: a meta-analysis of randomized controlled trials. Anesthesiology 2008;109(2):225–32.

27. Ebert TJ, Hall JE, Barney JA, et al. The effects of increasing plasma concentrations of dexmedetomidine in humans. Anesthesiology 2000;93(2):382–94.

28. Ornstein E, Young WL, Ostapkovich N, et al. Are all effects of esmolol equally rapid in onset? Anesth Analg 1995;81(2):297–300.

29. Talke P, Richardson CA, Scheinin M, et al. Postoperative pharmacokinetics and sympatholytic effects of dexmedetomidine. Anesth Analg 1997;85(5): 1136–42.

30. Ayoglu H, Yapakci O, Ugur MB, et al. Effectiveness of dexmedetomidine in reducing bleeding during septoplasty and tympanoplasty operations. J Clin Anesth 2008;20(6):437–41.

31. Durmus M, But AK, Dogan Z, et al. Effect of dexmedetomidine on bleeding during tympanoplasty or septorhinoplasty. Eur J Anaesthesiol 2007;24(5): 447–53.

32. Degoute CS, Ray MJ, Gueugniaud PY, et al. Remifentanil induces consistent and sustained controlled hypotension in children during middle ear surgery. Can J Anaesth 2003;50(3):270–6.

33. Richa F, Yazigi A, Sleilaty G, et al. Comparison between dexmedetomidine and remifentanil for controlled hypotension during tympanoplasty. Eur J Anaesthesiol 2008;25(5):369–74.

34. Lee LH, Irwin MG, Lui SK. Intraoperative remifentanil infusion does not increase postoperative opioid consumption compared with 70% nitrous oxide. Anesthesiology 2005;102(2):398–402.

35. Cai YR, Xu J, Chen LH, et al. Electromyographic monitoring of facial nerve under different levels of neuromuscular blockade during middle ear microsurgery. Chin Med J (Engl) 2009;122(3):311–4.

36. Honkavaara P, Saarnivaara L, Klemola UM. Prevention of nausea and vomiting with transdermal hyoscine in adults after middle ear surgery during general anaesthesia. Br J Anaesth 1994;73(6):763–6.

37. Usmani H, Siddiqui RA, Sharma SC, et al. Ondansetron and dexamethasone in middle ear procedures. Indian J Otolaryngol 2003;55(2):97–100.

38. Honkavaara P. Effect of ondansetron on nausea and vomiting after middle ear surgery during general anaesthesia. Br J Anaesth 1996;76(2):316–8.

39. Honkavaara P, Pyykko I. Surgeon's experience as a factor for emetic sequelae after middle ear surgery. Acta Anaesthesiol Scand 1998;42(9):1033–7.

40. Fujii Y, Toyooka H, Tanaka H. Prophylactic antiemetic therapy with a combination of granisetron and dexamethasone in patients undergoing middle ear surgery. Br J Anaesth 1998;81(5):754–6.

41. Fujii Y, Saitoh Y, Tanaka H, et al. Prophylactic therapy with combined granisetron and dexamethasone for the prevention of post-operative vomiting in children. Eur J Anaesthesiol 1999;16(6):376–9.

42. Gombar S, Kaur J, Kumar Gombar K, et al. Superior anti-emetic efficacy of granisetron-dexamethasone combination in children undergoing middle ear surgery. Acta Anaesthesiol Scand 2007;51(5):621–4.

43. Yeo J, Jung J, Ryu T, et al. Antiemetic efficacy of dexamethasone combined with midazolam after middle ear surgery. Otolaryngol Head Neck Surg 2009;141(6): 684–8.

44. Voronov P, Tobin MJ, Billings K, et al. Postoperative pain relief in infants undergoing myringotomy and tube placement: comparison of a novel regional anesthetic block to intranasal fentanyl–a pilot analysis. Paediatr Anaesth 2008; 18(12):1196–201.

Adult Laryngotracheal Surgery

Peng Xiao, MD*, Xiangwei (Shannon) Zhang, MD, MS

KEYWORDS

- Laryngeal carcinoma • Benign laryngeal neoplasm
- Preoperative assessment • Anesthesia management

The human larynx plays a pivotal role in airway protection, respiration, and phonation. The laryngeal disorders can be divided into two categories: benign lesions and malignant lesions. Most benign lesions are treatable with surgery and speech therapy, whereas the malignant lesions may require more invasive surgery as well as radiation and chemotherapy.

LARYNGEAL CARCINOMAS
Anatomy and Physiology

The larynx consists of a cartilaginous framework comprising the single thyroid, cricoid, and epiglottic cartilages and the paired arytenoids, corniculate, and cuneiform cartilages. The larynx is suspended from the hyoid bone by the thyrohyoid membrane. The vocal cords extend from the arytenoid cartilages posteriorly to the thyroid cartilage anteriorly. The primary function of the larynx involves phonation, respiration, and deglutition. Sound is produced following creation of subglottic pressure as expiration occurs against a closed glottis. The constrictive mechanism of the larynx results in an effective and rapid closure that prevents food, liquid, and other foreign material from entering the airway.

The larynx is divided into three anatomic regions: (1) supraglottis, which includes the lingual and laryngeal surface of the epiglottis, the aryepiglottic folds, the arytenoid cartilages, the false vocal folds, and the ventricle; (2) glottis, composed of true vocal cords and the anterior and posterior commissures; and (3) subglottis, which has no subcomponents and is the area of the larynx inferior to the glottis down to the inferior rim of the cricoid cartilage.

Supraglottic and glottic tumors are the most common, and subglottic carcinomas are rare. In the United States glottic carcinomas are the most common, accounting

Department of Anesthesiology, Massachusetts Eye and Ear Infirmary, Harvard Medical School, 243 Charles Street, Boston, MA 02114, USA
* Corresponding author.
E-mail address: Peng_Xiao@meei.harvard.edu

Anesthesiology Clin 28 (2010) 529–540
doi:10.1016/j.anclin.2010.07.010
1932-2275/10/$ – see front matter © 2010 Elsevier Inc. All rights reserved.

for 59%, supraglottic 40%, and subglottic 1%. This ratio does not hold worldwide. In Finland, for, example, supraglottic cancer outnumbers glottic cancer.

Epidemiology

Laryngeal carcinoma is the second most common malignancy of the head and neck. Each year, 11,000 new cases of laryngeal cancer will be diagnosed in the United States and 3600 cases with disease-specific mortality will be counted.[1] Incidence is higher in males than females (4:1); laryngeal cancer is most prevalent in patients 60 to 70 years old. The most frequently cited etiologic factors are heavy tobacco and alcohol use. More than 90% of laryngeal cancer is squamous cell carcinoma (SCC), and is directly linked to smoking and excessive alcohol use. Other risk factors (**Box 1**) that have been cited or identified are human papillomavirus (HPV), HPV 16,[2] neck irradiation, fruit and vegetable intake,[3] low body mass,[4] low socioeconomic status, laryngopharyngeal reflex, various occupational exposures to organic compounds, and toxic inhalation including wood dust, asbestos, and mustard gas. Laryngeal papillomavirus HPV results in laryngeal papillomatosis, which is usually benign, but subtypes 11 and 18 are known to degenerate to SCC. Patients with laryngeal cancer associated with HPV 16 infection have been found to have a better prognosis.[2]

Diagnosis and Evaluation

The symptoms of laryngeal carcinoma can be nonspecific. Common symptoms include weight loss, hoarseness, dysphagia, and odynophagia. In patients older than 50 years with a history of smoking and chronic alcohol use, hoarseness lasting longer than 3 weeks should warrant a referral to an otolaryngologist.

Further evaluation can include (1) complete head and neck examination, (2) visualization of the larynx by mirror and/or nasopharyngoscope, (3) direct laryngoscope and biopsy, and (4) computed tomography (CT)/magnetic resonance imaging or positron emission tomography. Except for advanced-stage tumors, most laryngeal cancers tend to remain confined to one anatomic site. Supraglottic tumors tend to remain above the true vocal cords.

Patients commonly present with persistent sore throat. Voice changes occur late in supraglottic tumors, and usually signify direct extension to the cricoarytenoid joint or paraglottic space involvement. Dysphagia and odynophagia are the most common symptoms and can suggest extension to the tongue base or to the hypopharynx.

Box 1
Risk factors for laryngeal carcinoma

1. Heavy tobacco and alcohol use

2. Human papilloma virus infection: HPV 16

3. Neck radiation therapy

4. Fruit and vegetable intake: inverse relation with the risk of head and neck cancer

5. Body mass: lower body mass index associated with increased risk of head and neck cancer

6. Low socioeconomic status

7. Laryngopharyngeal reflux

8. Occupational exposures to organic compounds, such as wood dust, asbestos, and mustard gas

Shortness of breath can be the presenting symptom with supraglottic tumors, as these are more likely to be present in association with cervical metastasis.

Usually confined around the region of the true vocal cords, glottic carcinomas are well-differentiated, slow-growing tumors. Due to the paucity of lymphatic drainage of the cords, glottic carcinomas often remain localized and have a less frequent rate of cervical metastasis.

Glottic tumors present very early with voice changes. Dysphagia and weight loss occur late in glottic tumors and are suggestive of vocal cord fixations, bulky disease, and extension to adjacent structures.

Preoperative Assessment

Preoperative evaluation of these patients must include evaluation of chronic medical conditions, dysfunction of multiple organ systems, and location and extent of laryngeal carcinomas.

Airway

Patients with laryngeal lesions are potentially difficult to ventilate and intubate. Patient symptoms and physical examination are indicators of potential difficulty. The history should focus on basic symptoms such as hoarseness or stridor as indicators of vocal cord involvement, while dyspnea and shortness of breath may occur as a result of mass effect or cord fixation. Prior surgery and radiation can cause anatomic distortion and dysfunction with swallowing, which may increase the risk of aspiration and hemorrhage. During the basic physical examination, the neck should be palpated for evidence of masses, tracheal deviation, and tissue plasticity. The most recent results of fiberoptic and mirror inspection by the surgeon should be obtained. CT scanning can be useful in assessing the extent of airway compromise. Once the potential problems with a patient's airway are identified, an approach can be devised for the maintenance of adequate airway control, and appropriate ventilation and intubation. Both the patient and the surgical team should be informed of the options discussed, including elective tracheostomy. Plans may need to include having a surgeon and instruments on hand for an emergency tracheostomy.

Pulmonary disease

Tobacco use is the one of the most important risk factors for laryngeal cancer. Eighty-five percent of laryngeal cancers can be attributed to tobacco and alcohol use. Current smokers have a 10- to 20-fold increased risk of laryngeal cancer compared with nonsmokers.[5] Risks have also been shown to decline following cessation of smoking. The heavy tobacco use in this patient population may lead to chronic obstructive pulmonary disease (COPD). Physiologic abnormalities seen in those with COPD include emphysema, chronic bronchitis, and chronic asthma. Pulmonary complications such as respiratory failure and pneumonia are more common in these patients. The identification and treatment of reversible components of pulmonary comorbidities are essential to improve the outcome. Treatment may include antibiotics for infection and exacerbation of chronic bronchitis, and bronchodilator therapy for reactive components of chronic airway disease.

Discontinuation of smoking decreases carboxyhemoglobin levels in 12 hours.[6] Mucous production, mucociliary clearance, and airway hyperactivity improve only after cessation of smoking for weeks or months. Preoperative smoking abstinence longer than 3 weeks improves wound healing in patients with reconstructive head and neck surgery.[7]

Alcohol and liver disease

The relationship of alcohol consumption to the relative risk is not clear. Most studies show that alcohol use is an independent and synergistic risk factor.[8] Chronic abuse is very common in this group of patients and may cause major systemic disturbances. These patients may have liver dysfunction and cirrhosis resulting in portal hypertension, splenomegaly, ascites, coagulopathy, encephalopathy, and hepatic failure. Cardiovascular issues include hyperdynamic increased cardiac output, increased intravascular volume, cardiomyopathy, congestive heart failure, and dysrhythmias. Pulmonary problems such as hypoxia secondary to extrinsic restrictive lung disease result from ascites-induced cephalad displacement of the diaphragm, right to left shunting, and pneumonia. Poor nutrition and vitamin deficiency may result in idiopathic macrocytic anemia. Gastritis, esophagitis, and varices may increase the risk of aspiration or gastrointestinal hemorrhage.

Anesthesia Consideration for Specific Surgical Procedures

The treatment of laryngeal cancer has evolved through three phases. The first focused on curing patients using radical surgical procedures, mainly by total laryngectomy. The second phase attempted to preserve the voice by use of oncological principles. The final and current phase is of organ-sparing protocols by using a combination of radiation, chemotherapy, and surgery. At present the overall five-year cure rate of survival for patients with laryngeal cancer is almost 70%.[9] The options for the treatment also depend on the stage of laryngeal cancer; early-stage laryngeal cancer can be treated with either surgery or radiation with the intent to preserve the larynx, whereas advanced-stage laryngeal cancer may require total laryngectomy.

Transoral Resection with Microlaryngoscopy

The first reported transoral excision of early glottic cancer is credited to Fraenkel in 1886.[10] This procedure was performed using mirror-guided removal of the tumor. Kirstein then introduced the first direct laryngoscope in 1895.[11] This early direct laryngoscope resembles a tongue depressor, but allowed for a direct visualization of laryngopharynx. The concept of direct laryngoscopy led to a development of various suspension laryngoscopes.[12]

Microlaryngoscopes use a suspension laryngoscope in conjunction with an operating microscope.[13] This innovation enhanced transoral laryngeal surgery because it provided excellent illumination, high-power magnification, and a three dimensional stereoscopic field of vision. Nowadays the microlaryngoscope is widely used for diagnosis of early laryngeal lesions, biopsy, and resection of vocal cord tumors. Surgical requirements include patient immobility and obtunded airway reflexes. An ideal anesthetic technique must provide a secure airway, adequate ventilation, no movement of vocal cords, and no risk of combustion, without time limitation for operative intervention. Depending on the procedure and surgeon preference, various anesthetic formulations can be used. Two basic techniques are most common: (1) general anesthesia with endotracheal intubation and (2) general anesthesia without intubation (the "tubeless technique").

General Anesthesia with Intubation

In patients without risk of airway obstruction, a standard intravenous or inhalational induction followed by placement of a small endotracheal tube will allow maximal view of the operative field. The procedures are usually brief and a short-acting muscle relaxant can be used. Remifentanil infusion in combination with inhalational anesthesia is very helpful to blunt the airway stimulation and minimize the inhalational anesthetic requirements.[14,15]

General Anesthesia Without Intubation: "Tubeless Technique"

Many surgeons prefer a tubeless technique for airway procedures, particularly when using laser resection of laryngeal papillomatosis. Intermittent apneic technique, jet ventilation, and tubeless spontaneous respiration are the most commonly used methods in the operating room. These techniques offer ideal operating conditions providing an unobstructed view of abducted immobile vocal cords. There is no combustible material in the airway, thus decreasing the risk of airway fire. The tubeless technique was first described by Talmage[16] and Judelman.[17]

Various intravenous medications were introduced later to avoid the use of inhalational agents. Propofol alone or in combination with remifentanil infusion are the most commonly used protocols. Propofol is an intravenous sedative and hypnotic agent with rapid onset. Remifentanil is a short acting mu-opioid analgesic that is very effective in controlling the airway stimulation during surgery. The combination of these two agents has excellent synergistic effects.

An apneic method involves ventilating the patient with an endotracheal tube and then intermittent removal of the ventilating tube for a few minutes to provide an unobstructed view for the surgeon. This sequence can be repeated as needed to finish the procedure. The disadvantages of this technique are that repetitive intubation and extubation may cause damage to the vocal cords and also prolong the procedure. The repeat intubation may also introduce laser debris and tumor tissue to the lower airway tract. The time period for the surgeon to operate is limited to only a few minutes for each sequence because the patient's oxygen saturation may decrease due to apnea.

Jet ventilation relies on air entrainment around the jet catheter to provide ventilation without endotracheal intubation. The surgeon has an unobstructed view of larynx. The disadvantages of this technique are the complications related to high pressure including pneumothorax, gastric distention, and dispersal of tumor tissue into the lungs. This technique should be used with caution in morbidly obese patients and patients with bullous emphysema.

Tubeless spontaneous respiration anesthesia is different from the other two tubeless methods. Spontaneous respiration anesthesia relies on maintenance of a patient's own respiration while keeping adequate depth of anesthesia with propofol and remifentanil infusion for the airway procedures. To keep this balance is often a challenge to the anesthesiologist. However, this technique provides adequate ventilation for the patient as well as an open view for the surgeon. The application of topical anesthesia to the larynx before suspension reduces vocal cord reactivity and decreases the risk of laryngospasm.[18,19]

Conservative Laryngectomy Surgery (Partial Laryngectomy)

The concept of partial laryngeal surgery is based on an understanding of the anatomy and embryology of the larynx. Fibroelastic membranes and ligaments divide the larynx into different compartments and the connective tissues resist the spread of tumor from one compartment to another. In the early stages of laryngeal cancer, it is not necessary to remove the entire larynx. Understanding the embryologic origin of the larynx helps to explain the difference in the clinical behavior between cancers arising from these laryngeal subsites. This evidence was elucidated by Tucker and Smith,[20] who studied whole organ sections at various stages of fetal development. Pressman[21] performed injection studies on the larynx with various radioisotopes and dyes in order to understand the anatomy of larynx and the spread of cancer within the larynx.

Hemilaryngectomy is the removal of one vertical half of the larynx. Appropriate tumors for this surgery are those with subglottic extension less than 1 cm below the true vocal cords, unilateral involvement, and no cartilage or extralaryngeal soft tissue involvement.

Supraglottic laryngectomy is the removal of the supraglottis or the upper part of the larynx. This procedure can be performed endoscopically using carbon dioxide laser or a standard open approach. Total laryngectomy is indicated when the tumor invades beyond the local laryngeal boundaries. In general, the larynx is removed from the hyoid bone to a few centimeters below the tumor margin including thyroid, cricoid cartilages, and possibly some upper tracheal rings. An en bloc dissection may be required for more extensive disease. The first successful total laryngectomy was performed by Enrico Bottini in 1874.[22] The early total laryngectomies were generally disastrous, with hemorrhage, sepsis, mediastinitis, pneumonia, and death. Pneumonia frequently developed after this operation because of the lack of separation of the aerodigestive tract. Solis-Cohen in the United States and Gluck in Europe were the first to develop techniques of total laryngectomy that separated the airway from the digestive tract.[23] With the advances in anesthesia and postoperative intensive care, the operative mortality rate dropped from 50% in late nineteenth century to 1% to 3% in the early twentieth century.[24]

Total Laryngopharyngectomy with Reconstruction

When tumors involve both the larynx and hypopharynx, laryngopharyngectomy is required. The procedure requires a more extensive operation involving surgical ablation of the larynx, hypopharynx, and upper cervical esophagus. Repair of the resulting defect may require transposition of tissue or the introduction of free vascularized tissue. The methods used in reconstructing laryngopharyngectomy defects have evolved over past decades. In the 1940s Wooky used anterior cervical skin as a graft to form a pharyngeal conduit. The deltopectoral transposition flap was used in the 1960s. Gastric pull-up and colonic transposition flaps were used in the 1970s. Since then myocutaneous flaps have been used to close partial laryngopharyngectomy defects. More recently, other techniques such as radial forearm flap, lateral thigh flap, and scapular fasciocutaneous flap have became popular. Since the early 1980s, the use of tracheoesophageal prostheses in patients with total laryngectomy has influenced the surgeon to favor stiffer tissue flaps over visceral flaps.[25]

Anesthesia Management for Free Flap Reconstruction Procedures

The success rate of free flap reconstruction can be influenced by many factors. Although the successful free flap procedure depends mainly on the skills of the surgeon, anesthesiologists also play an important role in improving the success rate of the free flap transfer by controlling the systemic blood pressure, blood volume, and local blood flow. The regional blood flow can be compromised by hypothermia, decreased cardiac output, and vasospasm from surgical stimulation. The changes in blood pressure, ventilation settings, and use of different anesthetic agents as well as vasoactive drugs can all affect the survival rate of free flaps.[26]

Hypovolemia is often associated with chronic hypertension due to the persistent vessel constriction. Preoperative fasting, inadequate intake, vomiting, and diarrhea are the common causes of preoperative hypovolemia. The inhalational and intravenous anesthetics can all cause vasodilatation and further decrease the effective blood volume. The blood flow in the free flap tissue has only about half of the pretransfer values even with patent arterial-venous anastomoses. Any further decrease in the blood flow may cause ischemia of the flap. One of the methods to improve the regional blood flow is to obtain a hyperdynamic circulation. It is believed that by fluid loading, cardiac output increases because of venous return augmentation and regional blood flow, and oxygen transport can be improved.[26] Fluid loading can also result in hemodilution and decrease the blood viscosity, and thereby further improve the cardiac output and microcirculations.

Alternatively, isovolemic hemodilution may be used to improve the microcirculation. Gao and colleagues[27] used a hemodilution technique in their 30 free flap patients during the procedure and five days postoperatively, with a flap survival rate of 93.3%. A very low hematocrit is associated with bleeding because the erythrocytes contribute to the process of hemostasis. Thus a hematocrit of 30% to 35% is recommended for vascular microsurgery.

The great controversy over the choice of optimal fluid replacement in surgical patients continues. There are conflicting studies regarding colloids versus crystalloids for surgical patients. The ideal fluid used for plasma replacement during vascular microsurgery should not pass through the endothelium to cause edema. The free flap tissue has already suffered hypoxia for some time, and the lymphatic drainage has been cut off and is more sensitive to edema than normal tissues. There is consensus that colloid solutions have a longer intravascular half-life and require less total volume than crystalloid, and cause less peripheral tissue edema. The available colloids are dextran, albumin (5% or 25%), and hydroxyethyl starch (hetastarch).

Dextran is a water-soluble polymer synthesized by certain bacteria from sucrose. The most commonly used preparation has mean molecular weights of 40,000 and 70,000 Da. Dextran-40 is frequently used as a 10% solution, which is hyperoncotic. Dextran-70 is usually available in a 6% solution and is nearly iso-oncotic. Dextran-40 remains intravascular for only 2 to 4 hours and is used in microvascular surgery to prevent thromboembolism by decreasing blood viscosity. High molecular weight dextrans remain in the intravascular space for 12 hours. These agents are used for expansion of intravascular fluid volume. Dextran decreases platelet adhesiveness and depresses activity of factors V, VIII, and IX, especially when high molecular weight dextran is infused and the dose is greater than 1500 mL. Dextran is associated with allergic reactions. Low molecular weight dextran has less antigenic potential than high molecular weight dextran. Dextran solutions may induce rouleaux formation and therefore interfere with subsequent cross-matching of blood. The blood sample for cross-matching should be obtained before dextran infusion.

Hydroxyethyl starch is a complex polysaccharide (average molecular weight 450,000 Da) that is available in a 6% aqueous solution. In fact, hydroxyethyl starch and albumin expand intravascular fluid volume equally effectively. Hydroxyethyl starch is removed from the circulation by renal excretion and redistribution. The duration of volume expansion is approximately 24 hours, which is similar to that produced by albumin. The starch chains are broken down into smaller ones by serum amylase. Therefore, serum macroamylasemia may follow and may interfere with the diagnosis of pancreatitis in some patients. Hydroxyethyl starch has been associated with a prolongation of activated partial thromboplastin time, a decrease in the plasma concentration of factor VIII, and decreased platelet function that is independent of dose administration. New-generation hydroxyethyl starches were developed by changing the mean molecular weight, molar substitution, and C2/C6 ratio. Voluven is the waxy maize-derived third-generation hydroxyethyl starch with mean molecular weight of 130,000 Da. Westphal and colleagues[28,29] suggested in their recent review article that the new generation of hydroxyethyl starch has reduced side effects on coagulation process, less tissue accumulation, and no unfavorable effects on renal function. In fact, there are many unsolved issues. Other studies have reported that hydroxyethyl starch 130/40 has similar side effects to the "older" one,[30] and the debate over the synthetic colloids or hydroxyethyl starch over crystalloids will continue.

Optimal ventilation should be set to avoid both hypoventilation and hyperventilation. Hyperventilation with respiratory alkalosis is associated with a decrease in cardiac output and peripheral vasoconstriction. Hypoventilation with respiratory acidosis may produce myocardial dysfunction and hemodynamic deterioration. Both inhalational and intravenous anesthetic agents can depress myocardial contractility and decrease systemic blood pressure. However, studies have shown that inhalational anesthetic agents, when compared with propofol, could have a beneficial effect on microcirculation by decreasing the extravasation of plasma into the interstitial space and limiting tissue edema.[31] Inhalational anesthetic agents may reduce ischemia-reperfusion injury.[32,33] Temperature control is crucial during vascular microsurgery. Hypothermia is a major cause of peripheral vasoconstriction. Intravenous and inhalational anesthetics inhibit thermoregulation in a dose-dependent manner. Hypothermia also causes erythrocyte and platelet aggregation, increased plasma viscosity, and further decreases in peripheral blood flow. Prevention and treatment of hypothermia may be difficult in a prolonged procedure that exposes a large body surface area. Passive techniques including cotton blanket and sterile drapes are insufficient to prevent heat loss. Active techniques including forced-air convective warming, conductive circulating water mattresses, intravenous fluid warming, and airway heating and humidification are very effective. Prewarming of the operating room before induction is also valuable. The central and peripheral temperature should be monitored. The difference between the two temperatures should not be larger than 2°C. A high gradient may reflect low volume status or a decrease in cardiac output.

The choice of nondepolarizing muscle relaxant is usually dictated by its cardiovascular effect and duration of action. Pancuronium has proved to be a suitable relaxant, as arterial blood pressure is well maintained and a slight tachycardia is usually produced. Adequate postoperative analgesia is essential, as pain enhances peripheral vasoconstriction and the patient will become restless. A balanced technique with opiate and sedative is optimal.

Vasoactive drugs

Free flap tissues are completely denervated. During surgery, blood vessels with a diameter of between 1 and 4 mm are anastomosed. The arteries can be categorized as resistance vessels. Many factors can change the blood flow to the flap tissue. The systemic arterial pressure gradient across the transplanted free flap is the major determinant. A decrease in arterial vasoconstriction or increase in venous pressure from edema can all reduce the blood flow to the free flap. The effect of vasoactive medications on the blood flow of free flap tissues have been studied by many investigators. Cordeiro and colleagues[34] studied the effects of dopamine, dobutamine, and phenylephrine on the free flap pig model, and found that dopamine infusion at either high or low dose had no effect on the flap blood flow despite increasing cardiac output. Dobutamine infusion increased cardiac output and improved the flap blood flow. Similar results were obtained by Scholz and colleagues[35] on patients using a dobutamine infusion at 4 to 6 μg/kg/min. It was shown by Codeiro and colleagues that doses of 1.5 and 3 μg/kg/min infusion of phenylephrine decrease the flap blood flow, while Banic and colleagues[36] showed in a porcine model that phenylephrine at 1 μg/kg/min had no adverse effect on blood flow in free musculocutaneous flaps even with an increase of 30% in mean arterial pressure. Banic and colleagues also studied the effects of sodium nitroprusside on blood flow in the free flap in the same porcine model, showing a 30% decrease in mean arterial pressure and a 40% decrease in free flap flow. In contrast, Christopher and colleagues[37] have routinely used sodium nitroprusside infusion as a vasodilator therapy during microvascular anastomosis to promote peripheral blood flow and prevent vascular spasm. The infusion rate was controlled to produce only a moderate decrease in arterial blood pressure (no <100 mm Hg). Heart rate was supported with atropine or glycopyrrolate to more than 75 beats per minute. Any decrease in central venous pressure was corrected by fluid augmentation to prevent hypovolemia. Other pharmacologic agents have been tried on flap blood flow, with variable effect. Ichioka and colleagues[38] used intravenous amrinone infusion and showed no effect on the flap blood flow, though it may help to treat vasospasm when used topically.

BENIGN NEOPLASM OF THE LARYNX
New Trends in Treatment of Laryngeal Papillomatosis

Recurrent respiratory papillomatosis (RRP) is the most common benign neoplasm of the larynx. The incidence in the United States is two cases per 100,000 adults and 4.5 per 100,000 children.[39–41] Thus more than 10,000 Americans suffer from respiratory papillomas. RRP is a disease of viral origin that is caused by HPV types 6 and 11. Although some individuals can acquire the virus through intimate contact, it can be transmitted from mother to fetus. Laryngeal papillomatosis is not considered a sexually transmitted disease.

The primary treatment for RRP has been surgical ablation with microdebriders and carbon dioxide laser. However, the carbon dioxide laser has the potential to cause thermal damage to adjacent normal tissues, while cold microdebriders can lead to scarring and fibrosis. After Anderson and Parrish[40] reported precise treatment of the microvascular lesion with pulse dye laser, subsequent pulse dye lasers were used to treat laryngeal papillomatosis. By properly selecting the wavelength that is maximally absorbed by hemoglobin in the red blood vessels, the target can be preferentially injured without transferring a significant amount of energy to surrounding tissues. The 585-nm pulse dye laser is a fiber-based angiolytic, and was designed so that any damage it causes is only confined to the perivascular region while preserving the epithelial covering of the vocal cords. As compared with the 585-nm pulse dye laser, the KTP-532 laser provides enhanced selective photoangiolysis due to its pulse width being tunable. It increases the precision and speed of procedures while preserving the very dedicated epithelial layer of the vocal cords. The KTP laser can be delivered on a laser fiber much smaller than that of the pulse dye laser.

ANESTHESIA MANAGEMENT

Patients with laryngeal papilloma frequently have some degree of respiratory compromise. Airway assessment should be carefully done before induction of anesthesia. The choice of anesthetics depends on the technique of ventilation during surgery, which can be conducted either with or without an endotracheal tube. General anesthesia can be induced either by inhalational agents or intravenous agents. For those at risk of airway obstruction, a variety of laryngoscope blades, video laryngoscopes, rigid bronchoscopes, and a tracheostomy tray should be available in the operating room. Tracheostomy may be necessary in some cases, but should be avoided at all costs to prevent distal spread of viruses to the trachea or bronchi. The commonly used 50% mixtures of O_2/N_2O can produce explosive conditions in the open airway, given the combination of high-intensity thermal beam and combustible material such as, endotracheal tubes, sponges, drapes, and anesthesia circuits. Nontarget tissue should be protected by layers of wet gauze. Safety goggles should be worn by health care providers. With the advancement of the new technology, selected adult patients with laryngeal papilloma can be treated in the office. The pulse dye laser can be used in the office through a flexible laryngoscope, without sedation or anesthesia.

ADJUVANT THERAPY

Although surgical removal of papillomatosis is very effective, no surgical intervention can prevent recurrence. Interferon-α, ribavirin, and indole-3-carbinol have all been used to treat virus infection with varying degrees of success. Cidofovir, an antiviral agent, has recently gained popularity but it can cause sustained permanent hoarseness. The vascularity of papillomas is a very important factor for its rapid recurrence. Vascular endothelial growth factor (VEGF) initiates a cascade of intracellular signal transduction pathways for the formation of new vessels. There is evidence that VEGF plays an important role in the pathogenesis of RRP.

Bevacizumab (Avastin) is a humanized monoclonal antibody that binds to VEGF and inhibits its angiogenic effects. It has been used to treat variety of metastatic malignant tumors. Avastin has also been used as a local injection to inhibit angiogenic processes such as macular degeneration.

A pilot study was done by Zeitels and colleagues[41] using sublesional injection of Avastin at the time of angiolytic laser surgery. All ten patients had a greater than 90% reduction in recurrence. Although a larger patient cohort and multi-institutional studies are required, the study provides a new avenue for research regarding adjuvant treatment of RRP.

REFERENCES

1. American Cancer Society. Cancer factor and figures 2007.
2. Curado MP, Hashible M. Recent changes in the epidemiology of head and neck cancer. Curr Opin Oncol 2009;21(3):201–5.
3. Freeman ND, Park Y, Subar AF, et al. Fruit and vegetable intake and head and neck cancer risk in a large United States prospective cohort study. Int J Cancer 2008;122:2330–6.
4. Peter ES, Luckett BG, Applebaum KM, et al. Dairy products, leanness, and head and neck squamous cell carcinoma. Head Neck 2008;30:1193–205.
5. Bosrtti C, Garavello W, Gallus S, et al. Effect of smoking cessation on the risk of laryngeal cancer: an overview of published studies. Oral Oncol 2006;42(9): 866–72.
6. Egan TD, Wong KC. Perioperative smoking cessation and anesthesia: a review. J Clin Anesth 1992;4:63–72.
7. Kuri M, Masashi M, Hideo T, et al. Determination of the duration of preoperative smoking cessation to improve wound healing after head and neck surgery. Anesthesiology 2005;102:892–6.
8. Sadir M, Mcmahon J, Parker A. Laryngeal dysplasia: etiology and molecular biology. J Laryngol Otol 2006;120(3):170–7.
9. American Cancer Society. Cancer factor and figures 2006.
10. Fraenkel B. First healing of laryngeal cancer taken out through the natural passages. Arch Klin Chir 1886;12:283–386.
11. Kirstein A. [Autoskopie des Larynx und der Trachea.] Arch Laryngol Rhinol 1895; 3:156–64 [in German].

12. Killian G. [Die Schwebelaryngoskopie.] Arch Laryngol Rhinol 1912;26:277–317 [in German].

13. Scalo AN, Shipman WF, Tabb HG. Microscopic suspension laryngoscopy. Ann Otol Rhinol Laryngol 1960;69:1134–8.

14. Burkle H, Dunbar S, Van AH. Remifentanil: a novel, short-acting, mu-opioid. Anesth Analg 1996;83:646–51.

15. Weisberger EC, Miner JD. Apneic anesthesia for improved endoscopic removal of laryngeal papillomata. Laryngoscope 1988;98:693–7.

16. Talmage EA. Endotracheal tube is not necessary for laryngeal microsurgery. Anesthesiology 1981;55:382.

17. Judelman H. Anesthesia for laryngoscopy and microsurgery of larynx. S Afr Med J 1974;48:462–4.

18. Pelton DA, Daly M, Cooper MA, et al. Plasma lidocaine concentrations following topical aerosol application to the trachea and bronchi. Can Anaesth Soc J 1970;17:250–5.

19. Quintal MC, Cunningham MJ, Ferrari LR. Tubeless spontaneous respiration technique for pediatric microlaryngeal surgery. Arch Otolaryngol Head Neck Surg 1997;123(2):209–14.

20. Tucker GF Jr, Smith HR. A histological demonstration of the development of laryngeal connective tissue compartments. Trans Am Acad Ophthalmol Otolaryngol 1962;66:308–18.

21. Pressman JJ. Submucosal compartment of the larynx. Ann Otol Rhinol Laryngol 1956;65:766–71.

22. Alberti PW. Panel discussion: the historical development of laryngectomy, II. The evolution of laryngology and laryngectomy in the mid-19th century. Laryngoscope 1975;85:288–9.

23. Holinger PH. Panel discussion: the historical development of laryngectomy. V. A century of progress of laryngectomies in the Northern hemisphere. Laryngoscope 1975;85:322–32.

24. Ogura JH, Thawley SE. Surgery of the larynx, otolaryngology. Philadelphia: WB Saunders; 1980. p. 2528–88.

25. Juarbe C. Overview of results with tracheoesophageal puncture after total laryngectomy. Bol Asoc Med P R 1989;81(11):455–7.

26. Sigurdsson GH, Thomson D. Anesthesia and microvascular surgery; clinical practice and research. Eur J Anaesthesiol 1995;12:101–2.

27. Gao Q, Zhou G, Chen G, et al. Application of hemodilution in microsurgical free flap transplantation. Microsurgery 1996;17:487–90.

28. Westphal M, James MFM, Kozek-Langenecker S, et al. Hydroxyethyl starches: different products—different effects. Anesthesiology 2009;111:187–202.

29. Jungheinrich C, Scharpf R, Wargenau M, et al. The pharmacokinetics and tolerability of an intravenous infusion of the new hydroxyethyl starch 130/0.4 (6% 500 ml) in mild-to-severe renal impairment. Anesth Analg 2009;95:544–51.

30. Reinhart K, Hartog CS, Brunkhorst FM. Hydroxyethyl starch: plus ca change, plus c'est la meme chose. Anesthesiology 2010;112:756–66.

31. Bruegger D, Bauer A, Finsterer U, et al. Microvascular changes during anesthesia: sevoflurane compared with propofol. Acta Anaesthesiol Scand 2002;46:481–7.

32. Lucchinetti E, Ambrosio S, Herrmann P, et al. Sevoflurane inhalation at sedative concentrations provides endothelial protection against ischemia-reperfusion injury in humans. Anesthesiology 2007;106:262–8.

33. Piriou V, Chiari P, Lhuillier F, et al. Pharmacological preconditioning: comparison of desflurane, sevoflurane, isoflurane and halothane in rabbit myocardium. Br J Anaesth 2002;89:486–91.

34. Cordeiro PG, Santamaria E, Hu QY, et al. Effects of vasoactive medications on the blood flow of island musculocutaneous flaps in swine. Ann Plast Surg 1997; 39:524–31.
35. Scholz A, Pugh S, Fardy M, et al. The effect of dobutamine on blood flow of free tissue transfer flaps during head and neck reconstructive surgery. Anaesthesia 2009;64:1089–93.
36. Banic A, Krejci V, Erni D, et al. Effects of sodium nitroprusside and phenylephrine on blood flow in free musculocutaneous flaps during general anesthesia. Anesthesiology 1999;90(1):147–55.
37. Christopher, Cox RG, Mayou BJ, et al. The role of anesthetic management in enhancing peripheral blood flow in patients undergoing free flap transfer. Ann R Coll Surg Engl 1985;67:177–9.
38. Ichioka S, Nakatsuka T, Ohura N, et al. Clinical use of amrinone in reconstructive surgery. Plast Reconstr Surg 2001;108:1931–7.
39. Derkay CS. Task force in recurrent respiratory papillomas. Arch Otolaryngol Head Neck Surg 1995;121:1386–91.
40. Anderson RR, Parrish JA. Microvasculature can be selectively damaged using dye lasers: a basic theory and experimental evidence in human skin. Lasers Surg Med 1981;1:263–76.
41. Zeitels SM, Lopez-Guerra G, Burns JA, et al. Microlaryngoscopic and office-based injection of bevacizumab (Avastin) to enhance 532-nm pulsed KTP laser treatment of glottal papillomatosis. Ann Otol Rhinol Laryngol Suppl 2009; 118(9 Suppl):2–13.

Applications of Ultrasonography in ENT: Airway Assessment and Nerve Blockade

James S. Green, MBBS, FRCA[a], Ban C.H. Tsui, MD, FRCPC[a,b],*

KEYWORDS

• Ultrasound • Airway • Regional • Anesthesia • ENT

The use of ultrasound imaging in anesthetic practice is becoming more widely adopted. It is currently used in many centers to facilitate vascular access and regional anesthesia in addition to the traditional role of diagnostic imaging. Using real-time ultrasonography, one can guide the needle directly toward the target (nerve for regional anesthesia, or vessel for vascular access) under visualization. Ultrasonography may help the clinician to avoid critical structures in the path of the needle, therefore potentially improving success while reducing complications. The use of ultrasonography in regional anesthesia has the additional benefit of allowing visualization of accurate distribution of local anesthetic.[1] Recent reports involving sonography of both the neck[2] and the upper airway[3] demonstrate its clinical potential at these anatomic locations.

As time progresses it is important to regularly review areas of ultrasound practice. In this review, the authors explore the use of ultrasonography in ear, nose, and throat (ENT) surgery and also illustrate, together with drawings of relevant regional anatomy, correct probe placement with corresponding ultrasound images. In particular, the use of ultrasonography for airway assessment and nerve blocks of the head and neck is encouraging. While much of the work in these areas is

Funding support: B.C.H.T. is supported by a Clinical Scholar Award from Alberta Heritage Foundation for Medical Research, Edmonton, Alberta, Canada, and a Career Scientist Award from the Canadian Anesthesiologists' Society/Abbott Laboratories, Toronto, Ontario, Canada.
Disclosure: The authors have nothing to disclose.
[a] Department of Anesthesiology and Pain Medicine, University of Alberta, 8-120 Clinical Sciences Building, Edmonton, Alberta, Canada T6G 2G3
[b] Department of Anesthesiology and Pain Medicine and Regional Anesthesia and Acute Pain Service, University of Alberta, 8440 112 Street NW, Edmonton, Alberta, Canada T6G 2B7
* Corresponding author. Department of Anesthesiology and Pain Medicine, University of Alberta, 8-120 Clinical Sciences Building, Edmonton, Alberta, Canada T6G 2G3.
E-mail address: btsui@ualberta.ca

Anesthesiology Clin 28 (2010) 541–553
doi:10.1016/j.anclin.2010.07.012
1932-2275/10/$ – see front matter © 2010 Elsevier Inc. All rights reserved.

preliminary, the authors attempt to answer pertinent questions such as: Does the use of ultrasonography have the potential to increase the sensitivity and specificity for prediction of difficult airway? Could it offer assistance for airway procedures such as percutaneous tracheostomy and awake fiberoptic intubation? Can the success and safety of regional anesthesia of the head and neck be improved with ultrasonography? And will the use of ultrasonography offer tangible clinical benefit in these areas that can be exploited in day-to-day clinical practice by the majority of anesthesiologists?

ULTRASONOGRAPHY IN AIRWAY ASSESSMENT AND MANAGEMENT
Percutaneous Tracheostomy

Percutaneous tracheostomy is frequently performed in the intensive care unit (ICU) setting. Many complications have been reported, including hemorrhage from local vessels and tracheal stenosis due to cranial placement of the tracheostomy.[4] The use of ultrasonography allows avoidance of vascular structures,[4,5] identification of the midline,[4,5] and identification of tracheal rings to avoid high (cranial) placement, and lowers the risk of laryngotracheal stenosis.[4,6]

In one observational study, ultrasound images of the anterior neck were obtained from 50 volunteers.[4] The distance between the caudal border of the cricoid cartilage and the second tracheal ring was found to be variable across subjects (range 9.7–29.7 mm). Consequently, it was proposed that the use of ultrasonography could be useful in accurately identifying the second to third cervical level for tracheostomy. The sonoanatomy of a longitudinal view of the larynx and trachea has been previously described (**Fig. 1**).[7]

An autopsy study compared the use of "blind" versus ultrasound-guided percutaneous dilatational tracheostomy (PDT) in ICU patients.[6] In 5 of 15 (33%) patients from the blind group the tracheostomy tube was found to be placed between the cricoid cartilage and the first tracheal ring (cranial misplacement). Cranial misplacement was not seen in the 11 patients for whom ultrasound imaging was used, indicating that the use of ultrasonography may reduce or eliminate misplacement.

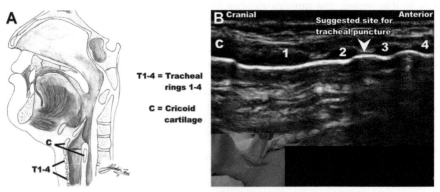

Fig. 1. (A) Regional anatomy and (B) ultrasound image (HFL38 6–13 MHz 38 mm footprint, Sonosite M-turbo; Bothell, WA) of cricoid cartilage and tracheal rings using midline longitudinal scanning plane at the level of the larynx on the anterior neck (probe placement in *inset*). The cricoid cartilage and the first 4 tracheal rings are seen, and the ultrasound shadow cast posteriorly from each of these rings aids with their identification. Overlying vessels, if identified due to their compressibility, will appear as hypoechoic structures, round to oval if seen in cross section or straight if seen longitudinally.

Sustic and Zupan[7] used ultrasound imaging in 30 patients prior to percutaneous tracheostomy to assist in identification of vessels proximal to the puncture site in addition to location of the midline and level of tracheal puncture. The tracheal midline, thyroid isthmus, and level for needle insertion were identifiable in all patients. Anterior jugular veins were identified and electively ligated in 15 patients. "Vulnerable" carotid or brachiocephalic arteries were identified in 4 patients.

Case reports on the use of ultrasonography for percutaneous tracheostomy following anterior cervical spine fixation[8] and in an obese patient[9] have indicated its potential usefulness in these challenging cases. The use of ultrasound imaging before insertion of percutaneous tracheostomy has the potential to improve clinical care by reducing the associated complications, but further studies are required for confirmation.

Visualization of the Epiglottis and Larynx

A sublingual approach for direct ultrasound visualization of the epiglottis was proposed by Tsui and Hui.[10] Further investigation revealed that the structure initially thought to be the epiglottis was in fact the hyoid bone.[11] Of the anatomic structures of interest, the epiglottis is suspended in air and the esophagus is posterior to the air-filled trachea (**Fig. 2**). Air is a poor ultrasound medium, appearing as a hyperechoic artifact that does not afford visualization of deeper structures.

Transverse and longitudinal transcutaneous imaging approaches have also been described for visualizing the epiglottis.[12,13] The appearance of the epiglottis can be captured through the hyothyroid window (between the hyoid bone and the thyroid cartilage) and its average anteroposterior thickness was found to be 2.49 $\pm$ 0.13 mm.[13] In transverse axis, the epiglottis appears as a curvilinear hypoechoic structure beneath an echogenic pre-epiglottic space and with dorsal acoustic shadowing.[13] For the longitudinal axis, Prasad and colleagues[12] use a parasagittal approach 2 cm lateral to the midline to identify the epiglottis cephalad and caudad to the hypoechoic mass of the hyoid bone. A hyperechogenicity adjacent to the epiglottis is described as the "mucocutaneous surface of the epiglottis due to the formation of the air-mucosa interface." This group has recently published an observational study to evaluate the feasibility of airway sonography (by an experienced

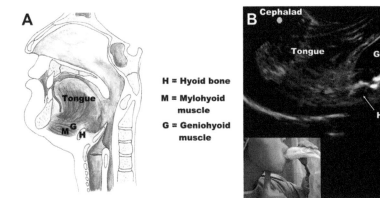

Fig. 2. Sublingual ultrasound imaging (C11 7–4 MHz curved, Sonosite M-turbo; Bothell, WA) fails to capture the epiglottis due to the presence of air, a poor ultrasound medium. As labeled in the regional anatomy drawing (A) and the image (B), the hyoid bone and its functional musculature is clearly identified *arrows*.

sonographer) and to determine the optimal scanning technique.[3] Due to acoustic shadowing from the hyoid bone, a parasagittal view of the epiglottis was only obtained by 71% of studied subjects. Singh and colleagues[3] used tongue protrusion and swallowing to confirm the identity of the epiglottis as a discrete mobile structure inferior to the base of the tongue. Reproducing such a clear view of the epiglottis in the parasagittal view can be challenging, as demonstrated by the authors' efforts at this technique (**Fig. 3**).[12] Also describing a parasagittal approach, Garel and colleagues[14] describe the epiglottis as appearing hyperechoic during laryngeal ultrasonography. Only the subhyoid portion was visible due to surrounding air obscuring the margin.

Epiglottal and pre-epiglottal edema (enlargement) due to pharyngolaryngeal infection has recently been diagnosed with ultrasonography.[15] A moderate increase in thickness of the epiglottis (3.2 mm as compared with 2.49 ± 0.13 mm found by Werner and colleagues[13]) was similar to the fiberoptic finding of moderate swelling. Ultrasonography to aid the diagnosis of epiglottitis may prove to be a useful tool for identification and management of this critical airway condition. The authors could not locate any trials evaluating the use of ultrasonography in epiglottitis for this review. The benefits of the use of ultrasonography in these situations—rapidity, noninvasiveness, and comfort—may speed its evaluation and clinical implementation.

Laryngeal ultrasonography has been used to investigate lymphangioma, laryngeal atresia, and papillomatosis, as well as subglottic stenosis and hemangioma.[14,16]

Prediction of Airway Difficulties

Ezri and colleagues[17] report on the use of ultrasonography to predict difficult intubation in obese patients. An abundance of pretracheal soft tissue (from the skin to the anterior aspect of the trachea) at the level of the vocal cords was found to be a predictor of difficult laryngoscopy. Patients in whom laryngoscopy was difficult had more pretracheal soft tissue (mean [SD] 28 [2.7] mm vs 17.5 [1.8] mm; $P<.001$) and a greater neck circumference (50 [3.8] vs 43.5 [2.2] cm; $P<.001$). Of note, 7 of 9

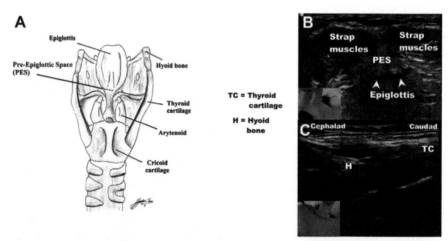

Fig. 3. (A) Relevant regional anatomy for visualizing the epiglottis (posterior view) and images captured (HFL38 6–13 MHz 38 mm footprint, Sonosite M-turbo; Bothell, WA) using (B) transverse and (C) parasagittal longitudinal scanning planes at the anterior aspect of the neck. The photos in the insets show the corresponding probe placement. Although a similar approach to that of Prasad and colleagues[12] was used here for illustrating the parasagittal view, the investigators had difficulty identifying the epiglottis in this view.

patients in whom laryngoscopy was difficult had a history of obstructive sleep apnea, which may have been associated with the greater neck circumference and increased pretracheal soft tissue. Four years later a group consisting of some of the same investigators published a study with similar methodology in the Unites States and reported conflicting results.[18]

Although Tsui and Hui[11] found sublingual ultrasonography to be of little value for assessing the epiglottis (see **Fig. 2**), they have observed that this imaging may have merit for predicting airway difficulties using the identification of the hyoid bone as a landmark.[19] In 1993, Chou and Wu[20] described a new predictive factor, hyomandibular distance, which may be increased in those with a difficult airway. Defined as the vertical distance between the upper margin of the hyoid bone and lower margin of the mandible, hyomandibular distance can be long for 2 reasons: a caudally displaced hyoid bone or a short mandibular ramus. Successful intubation by direct laryngoscopy requires alignment of the oral and pharyngeal axes followed by anterior displacement of the tongue and epiglottis. Caudal displacement of the hyoid bone may cause a larger proportion of the tongue to be situated in the hypopharynx.[21] Caudal displacement of the larynx would likely hinder the ability to visualize the hyoid bone. Its subsequent identification with sublingual ultrasonography may help predict difficult laryngoscopy and/or intubation. In a pilot study of 100 elective surgical patients, Hui and Tsui[19] (preliminary data reported) found that failure to identify the hyoid bone with sublingual ultrasonography predicted a laryngoscopic view of III or greater (11 patients having Grade III–IV view) with 72.7% sensitivity, 96.6% specificity, and 72.7% positive predictive value. These data show an improvement over other tests for predicting laryngoscopic view of greater than III: Mallampati score had 36.4% sensitivity, 87.6% specificity, and 26.7% positive predictive value, thyromental distance less than 6 cm had 9.1% sensitivity and 100% specificity, and decreased neck extension had 36.4% sensitivity and 88.8% specificity.

Confirmation of Correct Airway Device Placement

Ultrasonography has been used to confirm endotracheal tube placement in adults, both indirectly by visualization of diaphragmatic and pleural movement[22] and directly by visualization of a stylet or fluid-filled cuff.[23–25] In pediatrics, endotracheal tube placement has also been confirmed sonographically through visualization of the trachea and cords, with widening of the cords viewed on passage of the endotracheal tube.[26] Esophageal intubation was also seen in the paratracheal space in the same study. In cadavers, real-time transcricothyroid ultrasonography had high sensitivity (97%) and specificity (100%) for detecting esophageal endotracheal tube placement.[27] In another study, all of 5 patients with esophageal tube placement were identified as having such using transtracheal ultrasonography.[28] The correct placement of a double-lumen tube[29] and laryngeal mask airway (if filled with water)[25] have also been described.

Using longitudinal scanning, the appearance of endotracheal intubation has been described as a "snow storm" between 2 hyperechoic lines depicting the anterior and posterior laryngeal walls. This "snow storm" does not appear on esophageal intubation, and there may also be the appearance of movement posterior to the 2 laryngeal lines.[27] Static imaging after intubation has shown to be far inferior to dynamic (real-time) imaging for detecting esophageal intubation.[27] Transverse scanning with the probe placed at a 45° angle over the cricothyroid membrane results in an image of a curved thyroid cartilage superficially with the carotid arteries and internal jugular veins on either side.[28] Esophageal intubation produces a striking image with a clearly visible curved hyperechoic line with distal shadowing.

Current methods to confirm airway device placement include direct visualization of passage of the endotracheal tube between the vocal cords, end-tidal carbon dioxide monitoring, clinical examination, and bronchoscopy in the case of double-lumen tube placement. When combined, these methods are effective at detecting esophageal intubation and are readily accessible in the operating room. One disadvantage of relying on these methods is that gastric insufflation can occur before recognition of esophageal intubation. Ultrasonography could have a role in confirming endotracheal intubation, with the advantage of preventing gastric insufflation in the event of esophageal intubation; this may be particularly useful when passage of the endotracheal tube is not directly visualized (such as in Cormack Lehane Grade 3 or 4 view). Further research is required to fully evaluate the clinical impact of the routine use of ultrasonography for this indication.

Other Applications of Ultrasonography Related to the Airway

The presence of airway edema after oropharyngeal surgery may result in postextubation stridor. In an effort to overcome the limitations of the cuff-leak test, the ability of ultrasonography to predict postextubation stridor has been evaluated by using ultrasound-measured air-column widths.[30] In a study of 51 consecutive planned extubations, the air-leak volume (300 vs 25 mL) and air-column widths (6.4 vs 4.5 mm) were significantly less in patients with stridor (rate of 7.8%). These investigators placed the ultrasound probe transversely on the cricothyroid membrane while the patient's balloon cuff was both inflated and deflated. The air-column width was defined as the width of air that passed through the vocal cords, and this width noticeably enlarged on cuff deflation in patients who did not develop stridor.

Endobronchial ultrasonography has shown to be successful for distinguishing between compression of the airway and infiltration by tumor in patients with central thoracic malignancies,[31,32] for assessing expiratory airway collapse in chronic obstructive pulmonary disease and tracheomalacia,[33] and for assessing bronchial wall thickening in patients with asthma.[34] Endobronchial ultrasonography is not readily available for use by anesthesiologists in the majority of centers, limiting the scope for use. However, this is an area for future research to determine whether the use of endobronchial ultrasonography by anesthesiologists can direct management decisions and influence outcomes in situations with a critical airway problem.

Other uses of ultrasonography have been described, including the detection of a nonrecurrent laryngeal nerve in ENT patients,[35–37] and the detection of postoperative laryngeal nerve palsy using B-mode and color Doppler.[37,38]

APPLICATION OF ULTRASONOGRAPHY FOR NERVE BLOCKS IN ENT
Deep Cervical Plexus Block

Deep cervical plexus blocks have been used for anterior neck procedures such as awake carotid endarterectomy, lymph node biopsy, and plastic surgery.[39] Several ultrasound-guided approaches to the cervical plexus have been described.[2] An injection into the longus capitis at the level of C4 has shown to achieve blockade of the C2 to C5 nerve roots (located in a groove between the longus capitis and scalenus medius muscles) and of the sympathetic trunk (located on the anteromedial surface of the longus capitis muscle).[40] After performing an anatomic study in 28 cadavers, Usui and colleagues[40] determined that the injection position was localized to the site where a cranially directed ultrasound scan, initially focused on the scalenus anterior and longus capitis muscle at the level of C6, captured the point where the scalenus anterior muscle tapered off at either C3 or C4. Computed tomography showed that although confined to the muscle, the local anesthetic infiltrated into the neighboring nerve structures. An important finding from this article is that that the deep cervical plexus was not located in the interscalene groove, and that selective deep cervical plexus block can be performed in the groove between the longus capitis and scalenus medius (**Fig. 4**).

The cervical nerve roots travel in the sulcus between the anterior and posterior tubercles of the transverse processes, and course inferoposterior to the vertebral artery. The roots appear posterior to the anterior tubercles using a transverse view, but posterior to the vertebral artery using a longitudinal plane.[2] Identification of the vertebral artery and transverse processes of C2 to C4 allows cervical plexus block posterior to the artery.[2,39] Scanning caudally from the mastoid process, the level of the C2 transverse process and nerve root are identified through recognition of the loop that the vertebral artery makes as it travels between the foramen of C2 and C1. Subsequently, 3 injections may be performed between C1 and C4. Compared with blind landmark-based approaches, ultrasonography allows appraisal of both plexus depth (through location of the vertebral artery) and craniocaudal level (via the starting point of the arterial loop). **Fig. 5**[39] shows an image of the vertebral artery at the level of C2 to C3, and although the "loop" is not captured, the pulsatile artery is identified with ultrasound. It must be noted that these approaches are advanced ultrasound-guided techniques. Further evaluation of their safety is warranted prior to recommendation for widespread clinical use.

The use of ultrasound-guided high interscalene blocks and deep cervical plexus blocks to provide local anesthesia for carotid endarterectomy have also been described.[41,42] Using high-resolution ultrasonography, Roessel and colleagues[42] identified the upper portion (C4) of the brachial plexus, 1.5 ± 0.2 cm lateral to the common carotid artery, and although they used 20 mL of local anesthetic for the blocks as little as 5 mL was shown to surround the plexus. This indicates that ultrasonography may enable accurate placement of smaller doses of local anesthetic, thereby limiting the risk of systemic toxicity.

Kefalianakis and colleagues[41] reported high success with surgical anesthesia using ultrasound-guided block of the deep cervical plexus, combined with additional subcutaneous injection for superficial cervical plexus block and sedation. The local anesthetic for these deep blocks was injected between the scalenus anterior and sternocleidomastoid muscle at the level of the carotid bifurcation.

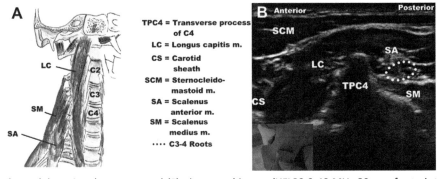

Fig. 4. (A) Regional anatomy and (B) ultrasound image (HFL38 6–13 MHz 38 mm footprint, Sonosite M-turbo; Bothell, WA) with the probe placed at the anterolateral position at the approximate level of C4. The photo in the inset shows corresponding probe placement. The longus capitis muscle is captured anterolateral to the carotid sheath.

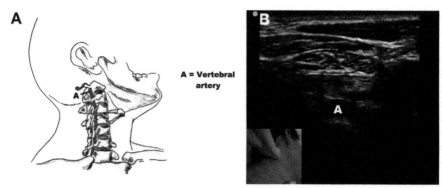

Fig. 5. (A) Regional anatomy and (B) ultrasound image (HFL38 6–13 MHz 38 mm footprint, Sonosite M-turbo; Bothell, WA) of the vertebral artery at the level of C2 to C3. The pulsatile artery was easily identified with ultrasonography.

Nerve Blocks for Awake Fiberoptic Intubation

At present, there is no ultrasound-guided nerve block specifically described for awake fiberoptic intubation. However, ultrasonography may be useful when performing several techniques for providing airway anesthesia. These methods include sensory nerve blockade or application of local anesthetics to the respiratory mucosa via cricothyroid needle puncture.

To provide anesthesia for the supraglottic larynx, the superior laryngeal nerve block can be used, while the cricothyroid injection has been shown to be effective for subglottic structures.[43] In clinical practice, the glossopharyngeal nerve block has also been shown to be effective for obtunding the gag reflex, although this approach is used less frequently. Because approaching the glossopharyngeal nerve via the styloid approach places the needle in close proximity to many blood vessels, it is anticipated that this risk may be reduced if direct visualization using ultrasound is used.

In a cadaveric study, the proximity of the superior laryngeal nerve to the greater cornu of the hyoid bone was demonstrated.[44] The mean distance from internal superior laryngeal nerve to the greater horn of the hyoid bone in a craniocaudal direction was found to be 2.4 mm. **Fig. 6** illustrates an image of the hyoid bone and the relevant anatomy for the superior laryngeal block, demonstrating that ultrasonography could facilitate deposition of local anesthetic at the superolateral aspect of the hyoid bone.

Ideally, the dual aims of airway anesthesia are to abolish sensory innervation and the afferent limbs of protective airway reflexes to facilitate endotracheal intubation. Nevertheless, the effectiveness of sensory nerve blocks has been compared with topical local anesthetic in spray and nebulized form.[45,46] Although patient comfort and hemodynamic stability may vary between the different approaches, intubating conditions are not any different.[45]

Alveolar Nerve Block

Ultrasonography for inferior alveolar nerve blockade for pulpal anesthesia (at the mandibular teeth) has been compared with the conventional technique in a randomized controlled study.[47] For this intraoral block, the transducer head with needle guide was placed on the medial aspect of the mandibular ramus to identify the mandibular ramus, the medial pterygoid and masseter muscles, and the inferior alveolar artery (using color Doppler). After localizing the artery, the needle was positioned in the guide

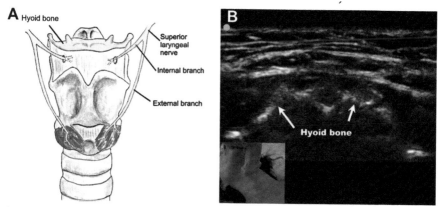

Fig. 6. (*A*) Regional anatomy and (*B*) ultrasound image (HFL38 6–13 MHz 38 mm footprint, Sonosite M-turbo; Bothell, WA) capturing hyoid bone, which may also be suitable for guidance of superior laryngeal nerve blockade (*arrows*).

and directed into the pterygomandibular space toward the neurovascular bundle. There was no difference in outcome between the ultrasound-guided and the blind technique, despite accurate placement of local anesthetic under imaging.

Superficial Trigeminal Nerve Blocks

Peripheral blocks of the terminal branches of the trigeminal nerve can be used for surgical repair of soft tissue injury of the face. Failure rates to achieve full anesthesia using traditional blocks of the trigeminal nerve have been reported in the region of 22%.[48] Infraorbital nerve blockade can be used to provide analgesia following surgery for cleft lip repair.[49] However, adult landmarks used to perform infraorbital nerve blocks are absent or difficult to palpate in the neonate. Facial foramina can be localized accurately and reliably using ultrasonography,[47,50] and this may provide an opportunity to improve success in these blocks. Recently, Tsui[50] described an ultrasound approach to locate the supraorbital, infraorbital, and mental foramina. Using a high-resolution, short-footprint linear transducer, a disruption of the continuity of bone in the vicinity of each foramen is used to identify the respective foramen (**Fig. 7**).

Greater Occipital Nerve Block

Local anesthetic block of the greater occipital nerve can be useful for certain neurosurgical procedures, for example, pin insertion for craniotomy, as well as for the treatment of chronic pain mediated by the greater occipital nerve. A recent cadaveric study compared 2 techniques of ultrasound guidance, using both the traditional block site and a selective approach at a proximal location where the nerve curls around the lower border of the obliquus capitis inferior muscle after emerging below the posterior arch of the atlas.[51] A transverse midline orientation is initially used to identify the external occipital protuberance. A caudal scan is used to identify the spinous process of C2 by its bifid appearance. A lateral rotation of the transducer is used to locate the obliquus capitis inferior muscle. The nerve is identified during its cranial course where it lies superficial to the muscle. Reported success of the simulated block, defined by spread of dye to the nerve, was 80% using the traditional landmarks compared with 100% with the new selective technique.

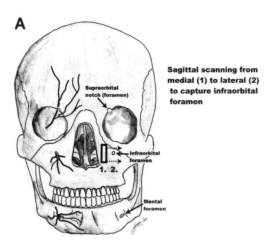

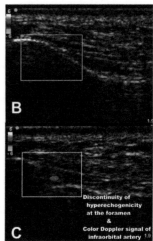

Fig. 7. (*A*) Skull with foramen and the respective nerves, and a representation of the scanning plane and direction (1. to 2.) used to localize the foramen as a discontinuation of the hyperechogenicity of the bone. Ultrasound images (HFL38 6–13 MHz 38 mm footprint, Sonosite M-turbo; Bothell, WA) are medial to the foramen (*B*) and at the foraminal position (*C*), where the discontinuation is clearly depicted and the artery is captured with color Doppler.

SUMMARY

The availability and use of ultrasonography in anesthesia is increasing in parallel with a diversity of indications for its use as technology improves. The clinical application of ultrasonography for the anesthesiologist practicing in the ENT field is in its infancy. This review of published literature shows that ultrasonography has the potential to increase the sensitivity and specificity for prediction of difficult airway, with promising evidence that failure to identify the hyoid bone with sublingual ultrasonography is predictive of a laryngoscopic view of III or greater. The use of ultrasonography to aid the diagnosis of epiglottitis may also prove to be clinically valuable in the management of this acute airway condition, and measurement of air column width to predict occurrence of postextubation stridor has obvious clinical appeal. There is great promise in using ultrasonography to aid safe placement of percutaneous tracheostomy, and location of the cricothyroid membrane and hyoid bone may be of value to assist anesthesia of the airway prior to awake fiberoptic intubation. There is also the possibility for improving success and safety of regional anesthesia of the head and neck through accurate needle placement and injection of local anesthetic. Although the potential for ultrasonography to improve clinical practice seems promising, the full extent of this will only become apparent over time.

Despite the potential for the use of ultrasonography in ENT, many ultrasound approaches described in this review are of academic interest and are not currently practical for routine use by the majority of practicing anesthesiologists or intensivists. Moreover, mastering the technical skills required to successfully interpret and use ultrasonography requires time and a detailed knowledge of the relevant anatomy. Further clinical studies are required to improve our understanding of this subject and to determine whether potential can be converted into tangible clinical benefit.

ACKNOWLEDGMENTS

The authors would like to thank Dr Derek Dillane (Assistant Professor) and Jennifer Pillay (Research Assistant), Department of Anesthesiology and Pain Medicine, University of Alberta, Edmonton, Alberta, Canada for their contributions, as well as Pillay's volunteering as a model for the ultrasound images and photographs. They also thank Jenkin Tsui (Student, Edmonton, Alberta, Canada) for creating the illustrations provided to highlight the relevant regional anatomy of the imaging approaches.

REFERENCES

1. Gray AT. Ultrasound-guided regional anesthesia: current state of the art. Anesthesiology 2006;104(2):368–73 [discussion].
2. Soeding P, Eizenberg N. Review article: anatomical considerations for ultrasound guidance for regional anesthesia of the neck and upper limb. Can J Anaesth 2009;56(7):518–33.
3. Singh M, Chin KJ, Chan VW, et al. Use of sonography for airway assessment: an observational study. J Ultrasound Med 2010;29(1):79–85.
4. Bertram S, Emshoff R, Norer B. Ultrasonographic anatomy of the anterior neck: implications for tracheostomy. J Oral Maxillofac Surg 1995;53(12):1420–4.
5. Hatfield A, Bodenham A. Portable ultrasonic scanning of the anterior neck before percutaneous dilatational tracheostomy. Anaesthesia 1999;54(7):660–3.
6. Sustic A, Kovac D, Zgaljardic Z, et al. Ultrasound-guided percutaneous dilatational tracheostomy: a safe method to avoid cranial misplacement of the tracheostomy tube. Intensive Care Med 2000;26(9):1379–81.
7. Sustic A, Zupan Z. Ultrasound guided tracheal puncture for non-surgical tracheostomy. Intensive Care Med 1998;24(1):92.
8. Sustic A, Zupan Z, Eskinja N, et al. Ultrasonographically guided percutaneous dilatational tracheostomy after anterior cervical spine fixation. Acta Anaesthesiol Scand 1999;43(10):1078–80.
9. Sustic A, Zupan Z, Antoncic I. Ultrasound-guided percutaneous dilatational tracheostomy with laryngeal mask airway control in a morbidly obese patient. J Clin Anesth 2004;16(2):121–3.
10. Tsui BC, Hui CM. Sublingual airway ultrasound imaging. Can J Anaesth 2008; 55(11):790–1.
11. Tsui BC, Hui CM. Challenges in sublingual airway ultrasound interpretation. Can J Anaesth 2009;56(5):393–4.
12. Prasad A, Singh M, Chan VW. Ultrasound imaging of the airway. Can J Anaesth 2009;56(11):868–9.
13. Werner SL, Jones RA, Emerman CL. Sonographic assessment of the epiglottis. Acad Emerg Med 2004;11(12):1358–60.
14. Garel C, Contencin P, Polonovski JM, et al. Laryngeal ultrasonography in infants and children: a new way of investigating. Normal and pathological findings. Int J Pediatr Otorhinolaryngol 1992;23(2):107–15.
15. Bektas F, Soyuncu S, Yigit O, et al. Sonographic diagnosis of epiglottal enlargement. Emerg Med J 2010;27(3):224–5.
16. Garel C, Hassan M, Legrand I, et al. Laryngeal ultrasonography in infants and children: pathological findings. Pediatr Radiol 1991;21(3):164–7.
17. Ezri T, Gewurtz G, Sessler DI, et al. Prediction of difficult laryngoscopy in obese patients by ultrasound quantification of anterior neck soft tissue. Anaesthesia 2003;58(11):1111–4.

18. Komatsu R, Sengupta P, Wadhwa A, et al. Ultrasound quantification of anterior soft tissue thickness fails to predict difficult laryngoscopy in obese patients. Anaesth Intensive Care 2007;35(1):32–7.
19. Hui C, Tsui BC. Sublingual ultrasound examination of the airway: a pilot study [abstract 613888]. Canadian Anesthesiologists' Society Annual Meeting 2009. Vancouver, June 26–30, 2009. Available at: http://cas.staging.swiftkicx.com/annual_meeting/abstracts_and_refresher/oral_competition08/pdfs/613888.pdf. Accessed July 21, 2010.
20. Chou HC, Wu TL. Mandibulohyoid distance in difficult laryngoscopy. Br J Anaesth 1993;71(3):335–9.
21. Chou HC, Wu TL. Rethinking the three axes alignment theory for direct laryngoscopy. Acta Anaesthesiol Scand 2001;45(2):261–2.
22. Sustic A. Role of ultrasound in the airway management of critically ill patients. Crit Care Med 2007;35(Suppl 5):S173–7.
23. Hatfield A, Bodenham A. Ultrasound: an emerging role in anaesthesia and intensive care. Br J Anaesth 1999;83(5):789–800.
24. Raphael DT, Conard FU III. Ultrasound confirmation of endotracheal tube placement. J Clin Ultrasound 1987;15(7):459–62.
25. Werner SL, Smith CE, Goldstein JR, et al. Pilot study to evaluate the accuracy of ultrasonography in confirming endotracheal tube placement. Ann Emerg Med 2007;49(1):75–80.
26. Marciniak B, Fayoux P, Hebrard A, et al. Airway management in children: ultrasonography assessment of tracheal intubation in real time? Anesth Analg 2009; 108(2):461–5.
27. Ma G, Davis DP, Schmitt J, et al. The sensitivity and specificity of transcricothyroid ultrasonography to confirm endotracheal tube placement in a cadaver model. J Emerg Med 2007;32(4):405–7.
28. Milling TJ, Jones M, Khan T, et al. Transtracheal 2-D ultrasound for identification of esophageal intubation. J Emerg Med 2007;32(4):409–14.
29. Sustic A, Miletic D, Protic A, et al. Can ultrasound be useful for predicting the size of a left double-lumen bronchial tube? Tracheal width as measured by ultrasonography versus computed tomography. J Clin Anesth 2008;20(4):247–52.
30. Ding LW, Wang HC, Wu HD, et al. Laryngeal ultrasound: a useful method in predicting post-extubation stridor. A pilot study. Eur Respir J 2006;27(2):384–9.
31. Bohme G. [Ultrasound diagnosis of the epiglottis]. HNO 1990;38(10):355–60 [in German].
32. Wakamatsu T, Tsushima K, Yasuo M, et al. Usefulness of preoperative endobronchial ultrasound for airway invasion around the trachea: esophageal cancer and thyroid cancer. Respiration 2006;73(5):651–7.
33. Murgu S, Kurimoto N, Colt H. Endobronchial ultrasound morphology of expiratory central airway collapse. Respirology 2008;13(2):315–9.
34. Shaw TJ, Wakely SL, Peebles CR, et al. Endobronchial ultrasound to assess airway wall thickening: validation in vitro and in vivo. Eur Respir J 2004;23(6):813–7.
35. Deveze A, Sebag F, Hubbard J, et al. Identification of patients with a non-recurrent inferior laryngeal nerve by duplex ultrasound of the brachiocephalic artery. Surg Radiol Anat 2003;25(3–4):263–9.
36. Huang SM, Wu TJ. Neck ultrasound for prediction of right nonrecurrent laryngeal nerve. Head Neck 2010;32(7):844–9.
37. Ooi LL. B-mode real-time ultrasound assessment of vocal cord function in recurrent laryngeal nerve palsy. Ann Acad Med Singap 1992;21(2):214–6.

38. Ooi LL, Chan HS, Soo KC. Color Doppler imaging for vocal cord palsy. Head Neck 1995;17(1):20–3.
39. Sandeman DJ, Griffiths MJ, Lennox AF. Ultrasound guided deep cervical plexus block. Anaesth Intensive Care 2006;34(2):240–4.
40. Usui Y, Kobayashi T, Kakinuma H, et al. An anatomical basis for blocking of the deep cervical plexus and cervical sympathetic tract using an ultrasound-guided technique. Anesth Analg 2010;110(3):964–8.
41. Kefalianakis F, Koeppel T, Geldner G, et al. [Carotid-surgery in ultrasound-guided anesthesia of the regio colli lateralis]. Anasthesiol Intensivmed Notfallmed Schmerzther 2005;40(10):576–81 [in German].
42. Roessel T, Wiessner D, Heller AR, et al. High-resolution ultrasound-guided high interscalene plexus block for carotid endarterectomy. Reg Anesth Pain Med 2007;32(3):247–53.
43. Tsui BC, Dillane D. Finucane. Neural blockade for surgery to the neck and head: clinical applications. In: Cousins MJ, Bridenbaugh PO, Carr D, et al, editors. Cousin and Bridenbaugh's neural blockade in clinical anesthesia and management of pain. 4th edition. Philadelphia: Lippincott Williams and Wilkins; 2008.
44. Furlan JC. Anatomical study applied to anesthetic block technique of the superior laryngeal nerve. Acta Anaesthesiol Scand 2002;46(2):199–202.
45. Kundra P, Kutralam S, Ravishankar M. Local anaesthesia for awake fibreoptic nasotracheal intubation. Acta Anaesthesiol Scand 2000;44(5):511–6.
46. Reasoner DK, Warner DS, Todd MM, et al. A comparison of anesthetic techniques for awake intubation in neurosurgical patients. J Neurosurg Anesthesiol 1995; 7(2):94–9.
47. Hannan L, Reader A, Nist R, et al. The use of ultrasound for guiding needle placement for inferior alveolar nerve blocks. Oral Surg Oral Med Oral Pathol Oral Radiol Endod 1999;87(6):658–65.
48. Pascal J, Charier D, Perret D, et al. Peripheral blocks of trigeminal nerve for facial soft-tissue surgery: learning from failures. Eur J Anaesthesiol 2005;22(6):480–2.
49. Prabhu KP, Wig J, Grewal S. Bilateral infraorbital nerve block is superior to peri-incisional infiltration for analgesia after repair of cleft lip. Scand J Plast Reconstr Surg Hand Surg 1999;33(1):83–7.
50. Tsui BC. Ultrasound imaging to localize foramina for superficial trigeminal nerve block. Can J Anaesth 2009;56(9):704–6.
51. Greher M, Moriggl B, Curatolo M, et al. Sonographic visualization and ultrasound-guided blockade of the greater occipital nerve: a comparison of two selective techniques confirmed by anatomical dissection. Br J Anaesth 2010;104(5): 637–42.

Anesthetic Considerations and Surgical Caveats for Awake Airway Surgery

Joshua H. Atkins, MD, PhD[a],*, Natasha Mirza, MD[b,c]

KEYWORDS

• Thyroplasty • Laryngeal surgery • Monitored anesthesia care
• Nebulization • Remifentanil • Dexmedetomidine
• Transnasal esophagoscopy • Laryngoplasty

The evolution of novel techniques for the treatment of laryngeal pathology has led to a significant expansion of the role of diagnostic assessment and the range of laryngeal procedures performed. Examples include vocal cord collagen injection, Gore-Tex thyroplasty, and laser ablation of localized laryngeal lesions. These procedures typically benefit from an anesthetic approach that diverges from a standard general endotracheal or laryngeal mask airway (LMA)-based inhalational anesthetic. The shared airway, need for intraoperative assessment of vocal cord function, risk of airway fire, and desire for rapid emergence and discharge are all important factors. In this article the authors undertake a collaborative anesthesia-surgical discussion of anesthetic management for airway procedures that are optimally performed with a spontaneously breathing, cooperative patient. An overview of pharmacologic approaches to airway anesthesia and cooperative sedation is presented, followed by a discussion of the surgical requirements and anesthetic goals of commonly performed procedures.

PATIENT EXPECTATIONS AND PREOPERATIVE PLANNING

The notion of participating in, or even remembering, a surgical procedure is anathema to the vast majority of patients. As such anesthetic planning for procedures that necessitate

The authors have no financial disclosures to make.
[a] Department of Anesthesiology and Critical Care, University of Pennsylvania, 680 Dulles Building, 3400 Spruce Street, Philadelphia, PA 19104, USA
[b] Department of Otorhinolaryngology, Head and Neck Surgery, University of Pennsylvania, 65 Silverstein, 3400 Spruce Street, Philadelphia, PA 19104, USA
[c] Penn Center for Voice and Swallowing, University of Pennsylvania, Philadelphia, PA, USA
* Corresponding author.
E-mail address: atkinsj@uphs.upenn.edu

patient participation or will be done under minimal sedation require the perioperative team to both set appropriate patient expectations and provide adequate education. Specifically, the patient should be counseled in detail as to what may be recalled, felt, seen, and heard from airway topicalization in the holding area to discharge home.

Most patients desire or expect complete amnesia of the perioperative experience. These expectations are not realistic in the awake airway surgery setting. Several studies in the setting of endoscopy for diagnostic gastroenterology procedures indicate that a large percentage of patients will refuse an elective procedure if done solely with local anesthetic.[1] Instead of amnesia the goals and benefits of analgesia, anxiolysis, and cooperation should be emphasized. Indeed a recent study demonstrated a high degree of patient satisfaction with the very unusual technique of cervical epidural and low-dose remifentanil sedation for complex tracheal resection.[2]

The authors find it helpful to review with the patient the advantages of "cooperative sedation," which include: (1) increased likelihood of optimal voice outcome during vocal cord surgery, (2) rapid postoperative mobilization and discharge home, (3) decreased potential for postoperative nausea and vomiting (PONV), and (4) avoidance of airway instrumentation (this is often the cause of the initial vocal cord dysfunction) and risk of associated airway management complications. Detailed preoperative discussion and agreement also affords the anesthesia team the benefit of not feeling compelled to aggressively titrate sedative hypnotics to the point of respiratory compromise simply toward the end goal of avoiding patient recall. It is also helpful to have a similar discussion with the entire perioperative team regarding the management of the anesthetic and the probability of intraoperative recall of events. Of course a subset of patients will refuse such an approach or be otherwise unsuited to sedation.

AIRWAY TOPICALIZATION: TECHNIQUE AND PHARMACOLOGIC CONSIDERATIONS

Effective topical anesthesia is a central component to any awake procedure in the airway. The ability to safely supplement inadequate local anesthetic–mediated suppression of airway reflexes with anesthetic agents such as opioids is limited.

A wide variety of approaches are well described for airway topicalization in preparation for bronchoscopy and awake fiberoptic intubation. Many of these approaches can be readily adapted to topicalization for airway surgery.[3] However, it is important to consider that many procedures are performed as elective ambulatory surgery. The approach to airway topicalization in a rapid-turnover, day surgery setting should emphasize consistency, cost effectiveness, efficiency, patient comfort, and patient satisfaction. For example, a patient who has not received preblock sedation may not readily tolerate needle-directed glossopharyngeal nerve block. Invasive blocks also use specialized equipment, need to be performed in the procedure suite, require practice for skill attainment, and risk hematoma formation. By contrast, nebulized lidocaine can be protocolized, delivered in the preprocedure holding area, uses equipment familiar to nursing staff and many patients, is noninvasive, and provides diffuse anesthetic delivery. Targeted individual nerve blocks remain an option in patients who cannot be adequately topicalized through noninvasive techniques. These blocks include glossopharyngeal, superior laryngeal, recurrent laryngeal/transtracheal, and cervical plexus, discussed in detail in a separate article by Jourdy and Kacker elsewhere in this issue.

NEBULIZED AND ATOMIZED LIDOCAINE

Nebulized lidocaine is a mainstay for airway topicalization in many procedure suites. Nebulizers, driven by oxygen, deliver small particles (typically 10–100 micrometer), and can thereby deliver aerosolized medications to both proximal and distal airways. The deposition of anesthetic in the oropharynx and tongue versus effective delivery to the trachea and distal airways is multifactorial. Important variables include particle diameter and density, functional residual capacity, tidal volume, flow rate, and viscosity of nebulization gas.[4] In general, mouth and throat deposition via oral breathing is less than nasal deposition via nose breathing. Patient anatomy (ie, mouth-throat length and volume) certainly plays a role in efficiency of delivery to the central airways, and substantial interindividual variability can be expected. Breathing pattern may be a relevant feature, and although normal tidal volume breathing is typically employed, some advocate periodic inspiration to inspiratory capacity with a breath hold. One limitation of nebulization is the time necessary to achieve adequate topicalization. This period is on the order of 10 to 20 minutes, and for most patients nebulization can be safely initiated in the preprocedure holding area. A range (1%–4%) of lidocaine concentrations has been studied.[5,6] More dilute concentrations trade decreased risk of overdose with longer duration to achieve adequate topicalization. A concentration of 2% lidocaine is a reasonable first approach, with 4% reserved for situations with limited available time or inadequate anesthesia. In most circumstances nebulization of 8 to 10 mL of the chosen local anesthetic solution will prove adequate and can be supplemented with atomization or gargling as described.

When attached to a mask, the nebulized local anesthetic can be delivered through the nasal passages as well. Nebulization can also be performed via a continuous or bilevel positive airway pressure circuit for inpatients with sleep apnea on noninvasive ventilation.

Lidocaine exhibits complex pharmacokinetics in the lung. Lung tissue acts as a lidocaine reservoir and may effect some degree of first-pass metabolism. Studies suggest that the plasma concentration of lidocaine after lidocaine nebulization is significantly lower than what would be calculated from intravenous injection of the same dose. In this way, nebulization is considered a safe, effective technique for airway anesthesia. An in vitro study by Tsui and Cunningham[7] demonstrated that 0.2 mL/min (8 mg/min) of 4% lidocaine was aerosolized at 4 L/min oxygen flows. Over a 15-minute period 120 mg of lidocaine would be delivered, which is well within the margin of safety for the average adult patient. Research in bronchoscopy patients suggests that this method is highly tolerable to most patients.[8] Kirkpatrick and colleagues[9] delivered nebulized lidocaine (4%, 6 L/min flow, 10 mL) to 10 healthy volunteers. These investigators found the gag reflex to be attenuated in all subjects, and serum lidocaine levels well below both toxic levels and the plasma concentration expected if the delivered 400 mg had been completely absorbed. Delayed peak of serum lidocaine concentration, as would occur with swallowing and gastric absorption, was not noted even after 120 minutes. Caution should be exercised in children and patients with significant liver dysfunction. One must always be alert to the possibility of local anesthetic toxicity. Symptoms include dizziness, tinnitus, disorientation, and signs such as arrhythmia, loss of consciousness, or seizure. Treatment is primarily supportive, with discontinuation of local anesthetic delivery, except in cases of cardiac toxicity for which additional treatment with intralipid bolus and infusion may be efficacious.[10]

After nebulization is completed, a curved laryngotracheal mucosal atomization device charged with lidocaine can be gradually advanced into the oropharynx with the tongue extended and the patient phonating. Topical anesthetic is sprayed into the back of the oropharynx and across the glottic inlet. The absence of a gag reflex during or after this procedure is associated with adequate topicalization of the oropharynx, glottic inlet, and proximal airway. Clinical data suggest that the combination of nebulization, atomization, and gargling without swallowing may be the most efficacious. In one study, despite the use of extremely high doses of lidocaine for gargling and nearing the "maximum" dose of lidocaine with nebulization and atomization, plasma lidocaine levels remained well below the toxic level in the healthy patients studied.[11] Gargling may be substituted with sucking on a tongue depressor coated with lidocaine gel (5%).

Topicalization of the nose can be achieved with nebulization. The use of oxymetazoline/phenylephrine spray is advocated to provide vasoconstriction, decongestion, and decreased risk of bleeding during nasal instrumentation. A field block of the nose (V2 branches of CN V, sphenopalatine ganglion of CN VII) can be accomplished by transnasal passage of pledgets soaked in lidocaine (2%–4%) or lidocaine-soaked cotton-tipped applicators for approximately 5 minutes. Applicators should be advanced gently to rest against the inferior, middle, and superior turbinates. This approach should be avoided in patients with a history of significant sinus surgery whose bony anatomy is abnormal, as passage of objects into the brain has been reported.[12]

After topicalization is completed, an intubating oral airway is placed into the oropharynx. Choice of oral airway intubation among Berman, Williams, and Ovassapian may be important, and has been reviewed in the context of fiberoptic intubation.[13] The shape and size of the intubating Berman airway are probably better suited to displacement of a large tongue from the posterior pharyngeal wall. However, the distal end of the intubating Berman airway, for example, intrudes into the vallecula and can be highly stimulating. The Ovassapian airway is relatively short and does not provide as much assistance with displacement of pharyngeal soft tissue, but has a lower profile and is adequate for simple bronchoscopic procedures. Frequently, a gentle jaw elevation at the time of bronchoscopy can serve to facilitate soft tissue displacement and glottic visualization in the sedated patient.

For transnasal procedures a lidocaine-coated nasal trumpet can be gently placed into the naris to provide broader anesthetic coverage. If left in place the nasal airway provides a smooth conduit for passage of the diagnostic scope and helps maintain airway patency in patients vulnerable to obstruction, even with minimal sedation. However, the nasal trumpet may trigger bleeding or interfere with vocalization or voice assessment in some patients. Care should be taken to identify patients at potentially increased risk of bleeding (eg, history of epistaxis, anticoagulant use, synthetic liver dysfunction, renal failure, thrombocytopenia).The authors typically perform these nasal blocks after sedation or analgesic infusion has been initiated.

THE COUGH REFLEX

Cough is a protective airway reflex mediated by bronchial, tracheal, laryngeal, and pulmonary afferent receptors. Cough is a major impediment to awake airway instrumentation or surgery. Intraoperative cough significantly disrupts surgical activity, may predispose to hematoma formation, may exacerbate glottic pathology or inflammation, and could promote vomiting if severe. Persistent intraoperative cough typically necessitates conversion to general anesthesia under suboptimal conditions.

The reader is referred to excellent recent reviews of cough neurophysiology and pharmacology by Canning and Chou.[14] Based on animal studies, afferent "cough receptors" have been categorized by anatomic location and functional physiology. In brief, the afferent limb of the cough reflex is principally mediated by tracheal/bronchial C-fibers of the vagus nerve and A-d mechanoreceptors in these locations. The subset of nerve fibers of principal interest for anesthesia of the upper airway is that located in the central airways including the tracheal, larynx, and carina. Such fibers are relatively sensitive to irritants and mechanical pressure as well as being vulnerable to topical anesthesia. Blocking activity of the recurrent laryngeal nerve, as opposed to the superior laryngeal nerve, appears to ablate much of the cough reflex mediated by proximal portions of the airway. General anesthesia has a complex, and not always inhibitory effect on these reflex pathways.

Lidocaine has broad and reliable antitussive activity that is primarily mediated by blockade of voltage-gated sodium channels at the level of the peripheral nerve terminal. Lidocaine nebulization is efficacious in reducing cough during airway instrumentation. Where lidocaine is not adequate or diffuse anesthesia of the oropharynx and airway is not necessary, pharmacologic supplementation can facilitate sedation and cough suppression.

Opioids are potent, well-studied suppressants of the cough reflex that act centrally on the nucleus tractus solitarius of the vagus nerve. Opioids also represent an effective adjunctive analgesia agent for use in combination with local anesthesia, ketamine, or dexmedetomidine. However, the pharmacodynamic profile of opioids, including the potential for respiratory depression and nausea, adds inherent challenges to anesthetic management. Opioids are discussed in the next section.

Dexmedetomidine (DEX) is a particularly useful sedative for achieving "cooperative" sedation. Applications for airway surgery are discussed in depth in a later section. In addition to sedation and hemodynamic stability, DEX has been shown to suppress cough response during emergence from general anesthesia and extubation.[15]

Various targets are under active clinical investigation as antitussive agents and could see wide application in anesthesia for airway procedures. One of the more intriguing approaches is work toward the development of lidocaine analogues that selectively target subtypes of voltage-gated sodium channels. In this way lidocaine toxicity, and specifically cardiac side effects, might be avoided.[16]

OPIOIDS, REMIFENTANIL, AND THE AIRWAY

Titratability to a defined end point is central to safe sedation during awake airway procedures. Moreover, if the agent used for titration has potential for serious, unwanted side effects, rapid reversibility is desirable. A variety of opioids is commonly used to blunt reflex responses to airway instrumentation. Important considerations in opioid selection include time to peak effect-site concentration, potency at the effect site, context-sensitive half-time, and elimination half-life.

The pharmacologic properties of remifentanil can be used to great advantage during sedation for procedures with rapidly varying levels of stimulus. Remifentanil potency at the μ-opioid receptor approximates that of fentanyl. Indeed both drugs equilibrate rapidly with the effect site (1–3 minutes), allowing bolus doses to be followed by noxious stimulus in short order. Remifentanil is rapidly metabolized in a liver-independent fashion by nonspecific plasma esterases. The elimination half-life of remifentanil is 3 minutes. More importantly, due to the mechanism of elimination, remifentanil is a context-insensitive opioid. The time for the plasma concentration of drug to drop by 50% (half-time) is for many drugs dependent on the duration (context) of infusion. This is especially true for fentanyl, which exhibits a dramatic increase in half-time with prolonged infusion.

All opioids depress respiration and interfere with cortical centers responsible for volitional control of respiration.[17] For awake airway surgery it is imperative that the effect-site concentration associated with apnea be greater than the level needed to blunt reflex response to noxious stimuli. Machata and colleagues[18] demonstrated that remifentanil infusions of 0.025 to 0.05 μg/kg/min allowed intubated postsurgical patients to tolerate an endotracheal tube while breathing spontaneously on pressure support ventilation. These doses were associated with light, cooperative sedation (Ramsay score of 3). Consistent with these findings, Gustorff and colleagues[19] found that remifentanil infusions at doses up to 0.1 μg/kg/min in the presence of mild noxious stimulus were compatible with maintenance of spontaneous ventilation in healthy, nonintubated volunteers. Xu and colleagues[20] used remifentanil (median effective dose 0.62 μg/kg bolus + 0.06 μg/kg/min) for sedated, topicalized fiberoptic intubation after topicalization and robust doses of midazolam (0.1 mg/kg). These doses of remifentanil can be predicted to result in bolus overshoot and then steady-state effect-site concentrations of less than 2 ng/mL (**Fig. 1**, blue line). A target concentration of 2 ng/mL is a reasonable goal. Modeling based on Minto kinetic models suggests that a bolus of 0.5 μg/kg over 1 minute followed by infusion at 0.1 μg/kg/min is a reasonable starting point (**Fig. 1**, green line). Subsequently the infusion can be titrated at (5) minute and 0.025- to 0.05-μg/kg/min intervals to achieve adequate sedation and reflex suppression. Infusion without bolus can also be considered but only if time is available for loading, as there will be a considerable delay in reaching the target effect-site concentration (**Fig. 1**, red line). In the authors' experience a mild diminution in respiratory rate from baseline, spontaneous eye closure, and ability to tolerate an oral airway or cotton-tipped nasal applicators are useful clinical end points to assist in guiding remifentanil titration.

Rapid effect-site equilibration and ultra-short half-life allow remifentanil to be titrated rapidly. Bolus dosing allows for ultra-rapid attainment of target plasma concentration but does not allow a gradual accumulation of arterial CO_2 to occur. Because opioids raise the apneic threshold, bolus dosing of remifentanil increases

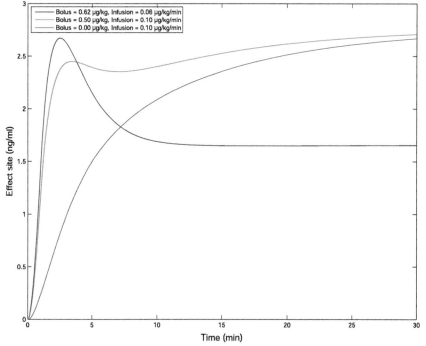

Fig. 1. Predicted effect-site concentrations of remifentanil after the indicated dosing regimen based on Minto kinetic models.

the risk of transient apnea. Thus, when bolus doses of remifentanil greater than 0.5 μg/kg are used, consideration should be given for preoxygenation with 100% oxygen via mask.

Capnometry (via cannula or mask) should be used in all patients receiving remifentanil infusion, as this is a more sensitive detector of hypoventilation than the pulse oximeter when supplemental oxygen is used.[21] Alternatively, the remifentanil infusion can be initiated with the patient breathing room air and being titrated slowly (every 3–5 minutes) until mild desaturation is noted, at which time supplemental oxygen is applied and the dose reduced by 25% to 50%. Following cessation of the infusion, the effect-site concentration will drop to clinically insignificant levels within several half-lives (9–15 minutes). Terminal elimination is also rapid and within the time period of standard recovery room stays; this allows the patient to experience rapid recovery and discharge without residual effects.

Two patient populations merit additional comment. Patients with obstructive sleep apnea (OSA) may be more susceptible to the respiratory depressant effects of opioids whereas chronic opioid users are more resistant. Bernards and colleagues[22] studied the effect of remifentanil infusion (0.075 μg/kg/min) on patients with moderate sleep apnea undergoing polysomnography. The results demonstrated, counterintuitively, an overall decrease in the frequency of obstructive events and an increase in arousals consistent with disruption of sleep architecture. However, the remifentanil group displayed an increased frequency of central (nonobstructive) apnea events supportive of the putative effects of opioids in modulating the activity of brainstem respiratory pattern generators. Thus, caution should be exercised when using remifentanil-based sedation in OSA patients for the possibility of sudden, central apnea. A subpopulation of patients with OSA is morbidly obese. Remifentanil pharmacokinetics in the obese population mirror those in leaner patients, and empiric dosing should be based on ideal or adjusted ideal body weight rather than total body weight.[23]

Patients on chronic opioid or methadone maintenance present a clinical conundrum in the perioperative period because of their altered responsiveness to these agents. Hay and colleagues[24] recently demonstrated that remifentanil is able to produce analgesia in awake volunteers on methadone maintenance therapy but at doses significantly higher (0.5–3.5 μg/kg/min) than used in opioid-naïve patients.

All opioids can be associated with PONV. Studies have not consistently found remifentanil, when used as a component of general anesthesia with propofol, to be associated with a statistically significant increase in risk of PONV compared with other opioids.[25–27] High-dose infusions of remifentanil (>1 μg/kg/min) were associated with nausea in healthy volunteers, and studies using remifentanil-midazolam combinations demonstrated an increased risk of PONV with "light" sedation.[28,29] Routine prophylaxis with a serotonin (5HT)-3 class medication before initiation of remifentanil infusion is a reasonable clinical intervention for these ambulatory procedures.

Benzodiazepines

Benzodiazepines, and particularly midazolam, are in widespread clinical use for procedural sedation. The primary pharmacologic effects of this class of drugs are anterograde amnesia and anxiolysis. Anxiolysis is the clinical end point for titration, and the patient can subjectively report it in reliable fashion. Midazolam is the only benzodiazepine with rapid effect-site equilibration, reasonable titratability, and short half-life. A potent, ultrashort-acting benzodiazepine, akin to remifentanil, would be highly desirable. Candidate drugs are under clinical development but none is available at present.[30]

Dose determination in the use of benzodiazepines to produce anterograde amnesia amounts to guesswork and clinical "experience." The dose-response curve for midazolam and amnesia in a given patient is not well defined and will be modified by the addition of other agents. Substantial pharmacodynamic variation can be expected and is unpredictable. This situation is an impractical one during airway surgery because amnesia accompanied by oversedation, agitation, or airway obstruction is unacceptable. Indeed, Williams and colleagues[31] studied the utility of aggressive midazolam dosing in a mainly elderly population presenting for bronchoscopy. These investigators found that even at a mean midazolam dose of 0.095 mg/kg, 3% of patients experienced some recall and more than 8% of patients required flumazenil reversal. A recent study of bronchoscopy under local anesthetic with midazolam versus propofol found that a similarly large midazolam dose in a younger population demonstrated slow recovery and risk of severe respiratory depression (eg, 2 patients required emergency intubation).[32]

The pharmacologic effects of midazolam, especially regarding hypnosis, are enhanced synergistically by α2-agonists and opioids,[33] which may lead to hypoxemia and apnea.[34] Indeed in some studies midazolam had an equivalent effect to propofol on reduction of airway tone and predisposition to airway collapse.[35] Drummond[36] demonstrated decreased muscle activity in the genioglossus and accessory muscles of respiration with low-dose (0.02 mg/kg) midazolam. These effects may be mediated by a γ-aminobutyric acid (GABA)-induced decrease in hypoglossal nerve output, or anesthetic-related suppression of pharyngeal dilators involved in the negative pressure reflex.[37] Another study found a relationship between head position and propensity for obstruction under midazolam sedation. There was a progressive propensity for inspiratory airflow limitation from 30° head-elevated position to the supine position that was attenuated by supine neck extension.[38] Systemically absorbed local anesthetic may also potentiate the effects of midazolam at doses used for deep sedation.[39] The addition of propofol to midazolam reduces midazolam clearance and distribution, and may increase midazolam plasma concentrations by as much as 25%.[40] The extent to which drug synergy will be demonstrated in an individual patient is again very unpredictable, as is the susceptibility of a given patient to upper airway collapse or obstruction. The addition of fentanyl to midazolam premedication may result in severe airway obstruction, attributable to diminished upper airway tone, which requires aggressive support and pharmacologic reversal with naloxone[41]; this is also true for remifentanil. However, remifentanil is more readily titrated and can be rapidly cleared in the event of overdose. A study of remifentanil versus remifentanil-midazolam sedation for ambulatory surgery found a combination of low-dose midazolam (1–2 mg) and low-dose remifentanil (1 μg/kg bolus then 0.05–0.1 μg/kg/min) to be safe, and relatively devoid of respiratory events.[29] However, airway surgery was not performed in this study and there was limited apparent benefit from the addition of midazolam. The midazolam-remifentanil cohort demonstrated a slightly greater tendency toward respiratory depression even with lower remifentanil doses. This result was consistent with that of an earlier study in which doses of midazolam greater than 2.0 mg with low-dose remifentanil infusion increased the propensity for oversedation.[28]

The authors do not intend to suggest that midazolam does not have a role in anesthesia for awake airway surgery. Rather, they wish to make the point that the use of midazolam in combination with other agents for airway surgery at common sedative doses to reach poorly defined end points may result in several undesirable outcomes: (1) the need for a respiratory intervention that may disrupt surgery (eg, higher oxygen, airway maneuver/device), (2) slower recovery, (3) recall despite attempted amnesia, and (4) risk of "atypical" reaction with agitation and need to convert to general anesthesia. In their practice the authors prefer to avoid benzodiazepines in patients predisposed to obstruction (morbidly obese, OSA) and otherwise use it in sparing doses (0.5–2.0 mg) for most patients. These doses in naïve patients will typically produce adequate anxiolysis. The dose-sparing effect of dexmedetomidine on midazolam pharmacodynamics has not been adequately delineated through isobolographic analysis or response-surface modeling. Functional magnetic resonance imaging is a promising approach toward understanding the neuropharmacology of amnestic agents used for sedation.[42]

Dexmedetomidine

Dexmedetomidine (DEX) is a novel agent in the armamentarium of sedatives. DEX is a highly selective, centrally acting α2-adrenoreceptor agonist that gained United Stated Food and Drug Administration approval for procedural sedation in 2009, but has evidenced considerable use in the past decade for the management of patients with precarious airways. An extensive review of studies of DEX usage in nonintubated patients was published recently.[43] DEX is used to great effect for "awake" craniotomy, a procedure that bears important similarities to awake airway surgery.[44] Sedation with DEX is notable for the ability to consistently achieve a state of anxiolysis and hypnosis with minimal respiratory depression. The term "cooperative sedation" is often used to describe the clinical state resulting from DEX. In a prospective, randomized study of 326 patients presenting for surgery under sedation, DEX reliably achieved this state with decreased need for opioid or benzodiazepine rescue compared with placebo.[45] Sedation with DEX phenotypically and neurobiologically resembles sleep more than sedation accomplished with midazolam, propofol, and other combinations. Patients tend to be asleep but readily arousable and yet can also be startled by sudden sounds or stimulation. Minute ventilation, tidal volume, and respiratory rate are preserved with DEX infusion. Patients "asleep" on DEX demonstrate increased minute ventilation and arousal with carbon dioxide challenge.[46] A study of the effects of DEX on a small cohort of healthy children undergoing magnetic resonance imaging with DEX sedation found that airway anteroposterior diameter, transverse diameter, and cross-sectional areas were minimally changed from baseline at doses used in routine clinical practice.[47] During DEX infusion an obstructed breathing pattern can occur in susceptible patients. In the authors' clinical experience the likelihood of airway obstruction is increased with the use of sedative adjuvants with respiratory depressant properties, such as midazolam or remifentanil. When used alone, DEX is associated with an unpredictable, and often negligible, degree of amnesia. A recent study in rats suggests that DEX-associated amnesia may be secondary to decreased processing of sensory input rather than direct blockade of memory consolidation.[48] As noted earlier, patient expectations to "not remember anything" should be suitably adjusted if DEX is to be used as a sole agent. A crossover study comparing DEX and midazolam for third molar extraction demonstrated that despite the fact that most patients recalled aspects of the procedure, satisfaction scores were high with DEX and better than with midazolam. In the midazolam group, 10% of patients administered 0.1 mg/kg demonstrated recall.[49] Amnestic synergy with small doses of midazolam likely occurs but dose responsiveness remains to be established. In a recent study of sedation for topicalized, fiberoptic intubation, DEX + low-dose midazolam (0.02 mg/kg) was associated with better conditions, fewer adverse events, and improved patient satisfaction compared with high-dose midazolam alone.[50]

Several pharmacokinetic and pharmacodynamic properties of DEX limit its routine use in outpatient surgery. The potent α2-agonist results in marked reduction of sympathetic tone, as commonly evidenced by bradycardia and moderate hypotension. The marked reduction in sympathetic output is problematic for patients with significant impairment of cardiac contractility or intrinsic conduction abnormalities. Bradycardia may be enhanced by the addition of remifentanil, but is typically moderated by intravenous administration of low-dose anticholinergic agents such as glycopyrrolate or atropine. Furthermore, the pharmacokinetics of DEX are such that (1) a loading dose should be administered slowly over a minimum of 10 minutes and (2) residual effects, including somnolence and hypotension, can persist for up to several hours after the end of infusion. These aspects may impair clinical efficiency, delay recovery, and extend postanesthesia care unit (PACU) stay. As such, DEX is not the optimal agent for brief, minimally invasive procedures in which both surgeon and patient desire ultrarapid recovery to baseline unless the technical aspects of the procedure merit its use.

The precise mechanism of DEX action in hypnosis and anxiolysis remains unknown. One hypothesis holds that DEX-mediated reduction of norepinephrine output by the locus coeruleus is the primary mechanism for sedative effects. Mice lacking α2A-adrenoceptors are immune to DEX sedation. However, recent data from Gilsbach and colleagues[51] reveal that transgenic mice in which α2-adrenoreceptors are expressed only in adrenergic cells were also immune to DEX-induced loss of the righting reflex. This result suggests that sedative effects may be mediated by α2A-receptors in nonadrenergic cells.

The sedative properties of benzodiazepines and the analgesic properties of opioids and ketamine are enhanced when used in conjunction with DEX.[52] If DEX is not used alone, sufficient relatively low doses of other agents can be added to support DEX sedation. A study of the combination of oral clonidine and morphine suggests that the addition of opioid to α2-mediated sedation does not produce synergy in respiratory depression.[53] A more recent study in healthy volunteers successfully induced similar depth of sedation with DEX/remifentanil and midazolam/remifentanil, but noted more potent electroencephalographic suppression with DEX despite identical Ramsay sedation scores.[54]

DEX is an excellent agent for use in "awake" vocal cord surgery such as Gore-Tex medialization thyroplasty, awake tracheostomy, and bronchoscopy. (See video at www.anesthesiology.theclinics.com.) As described in further detail later, the authors employ DEX with ketamine as the standard anesthetic for thyroplasty and awake tracheostomy. Advantages of DEX include: (1) potential to avoid supplemental oxygen and reduce risk of airway fire, (2) low likelihood of need for an airway intervention, (3) reliability in eliciting participation (eg, phonation) of patient at crucial times during surgery, and (4) simple dosing regimen with limited patient-to-patient variability. Published data on DEX use in airway surgery are limited; however, a case series of DEX use in various airway procedures was recently reported.[55]

Supplementary video related to this article can be found at DOI:10.1016/j.anclin. 2010.07.013.

Ketamine

Ketamine is an N-methyl-D-aspartic acid (NMDA) antagonist that has been in widespread clinical use for decades, both alone and in combination, to provide analgesia, general anesthesia, and sedation. Perceived advantages of ketamine include sympathetic stimulation, lack of respiratory depression, and some degree of intrinsic analgesia. As with DEX, the neural mechanisms by which ketamine exerts anesthetic effects are not precisely understood but relate to modulation of NMDA activity. During ketamine anesthesia functional residual capacity, minute ventilation, tidal volume, and ventilatory responsiveness to CO_2 challenge are largely maintained.[56] In one study of healthy volunteers, ketamine was shown to counteract alfentanil-induced hypoventilation via an increase in respiratory rate.[57] Ketamine may alter physiologic brainstem respiratory control via inhibition of pontine pneumotaxic centers, as evidenced by apneustic breathing patterns in animal studies. Airway protective reflexes and pharyngeal tone are largely preserved at sedative doses (1 mg/kg).[36]

Ketamine is seldom used as a sole agent, due to its potential psychedelic side effects that include unpleasant dreams and disturbing hallucinations in some patient populations. The risk of these effects is likely mitigated by dosing of ketamine after the administration of GABA agonists including propofol and benzodiazepines. The utility of DEX in reducing psychedelic side effects is not well studied, although a study from the Washington University School of Medicine is actively researching this question (http://clinicaltrials.gov/ct2/show/NCT00205712).

The authors' clinical experience with the combination of DEX and ketamine suggests that most patients still experience dream or trance-like states but rarely an overtly disturbing experience. Levanen and colleagues[58] compared fixed-dose midazolam and DEX premedication for ketamine/nitrous oxide based general anesthesia. In the postoperative questionnaire fewer patients in the DEX group reported central nervous system side effects (5% vs 55%) although the design of this study makes it difficult to extrapolate to intravenous ketamine-DEX sedation. Concomitant use of midazolam does not provide a guarantee against psychiatric effects, may contribute to respiratory depression events. In contrast, DEX is loaded according to a standard regimen (1 μg/kg over 10 minutes) for most patients and is titrated to induce sleep or maintenance of spontaneous eye closure.

The potential for untoward psychiatric effects in some studies also demonstrates a dose-dependent, threshold effect. Very low doses such as those commonly used for adjunctive or preemptive analgesia are believed to be relatively safe from the psychiatric perspective.[59] Midazolam premedication is frequently employed in an effort to modulate the psychiatric properties but is not necessarily effective.[60] The effect-site concentration needed to decrease psychedelic effects is unknown. Certain patient populations including those with established psychotic disease, history of hallucinogenic drug use, or severe emotional trauma may be at increased risk of unpleasant psychedelic effects.

Ketamine equilibrates rapidly with the effect site. The offset of ketamine is also relatively rapid, and use of a continuous infusion during sedation is optimal. Several dosing regimens for sedation and perioperative analgesia are described in the literature.[61] A bolus dose of 0.5 mg/kg is usually sufficient to induce dissociation during which time invasive procedures such as local injection at the surgical site, transtracheal block, or fiberoptic examination of the airway can be performed. In the authors' experience, when combined with DEX, maintenance with a continuous infusion of ketamine (3–10 μg/kg/min) provides additional analgesia and light hypnosis that is commonly compatible with intraoperative cooperation or is readily reversible after termination of infusion.

The combination of DEX and ketamine is an emerging anesthetic for surgical procedures under sedation in which additional analgesia and hypnosis is needed.[62–65] Examples include fiberoptic intubation, interventional pulmonology (eg, endobronchial ultrasonography, stenting), laryngoplasty, thyroplasty, esophagoscopy, transesophageal echocardiography, and cardiac catheterization. Ketamine can to some extent counteract the sympathetic depressant effects of DEX, is a respiratory stimulant, provides reliable hypnosis during injections of local, is readily titratable, and possesses intrinsic analgesic properties that may be enhanced by DEX. Pretreatment with glycopyrrolate can reduce the associated increase in secretions, and DEX itself is a mild antisialogogue.

SURGICAL PROCEDURES

Office-based laryngeal surgery has recently been reviewed.[66] The goal of this section is to discuss procedures done in an endoscopy suite model. The advantages of these procedures in this setting are an increase in patient cooperation during the procedure, the ability to monitor the voice during a surgical intervention, and rapid recovery.[67] In fact endoscopy procedures under modified anesthesia techniques offer increased safety and access for some patients deemed to have a "difficult airway." The assessment of the awake airway, including both the larynx and trachea, allows the surgeon to obtain a dynamic view when the patient is able to maintain spontaneous breathing and has less airway collapse. The newer endoscopes and high-definition monitoring systems have further refined these techniques.[68,69] For most of these techniques the patients do not require extensive preoperative testing, as the anesthetic is expected to have minimal hemodynamic impact. However, workup should be determined on a case-by-case basis and should adhere to local standards for office-based surgery and anesthesia. For the patient with anxiety for whom a procedure is not feasible without sedation, the described anesthetic approach offers a safe and convenient alternative to general anesthesia with intubation.

A focused primer on thyroplasty, esophagoscopy, bronchoscopy, and related laryngeal procedures is presented with a discussion on surgical needs as they relate to considerations.

Most procedures require topical anesthesia of the nasal passages and the oropharynx and hypopharynx and laryngeal inlet and vocal folds, as described earlier. A pediatric bronchoscope is typically used because it has a port for delivery of additional topical anesthetic directly onto the vocal folds if necessary. Although recovery is quick, the effects of the local anesthesia are generally longer lasting and can last for 60 to 90 minutes.

The following procedures are discussed:

1. Diagnostic endoscopies of larynx, trachea, and bronchi
2. Esophagoscopy
3. Laryngeal and tracheal stenosis
4. Laser laryngoscopy and bronchoscopy
5. Vocal fold injections for medialization
6. Esophagoscopy (both transnasal and per oral esophagoscopy)
7. Laryngotracheal biopsies
8. Transesophageal punctures
9. Gore-Tex medialization thyroplasty.

Diagnostic Endoscopies

Esophagoscopy in the office is a primary diagnostic tool for otolaryngologists.[70] Esophagoscopy comprises primarily office-based procedures conceptually done under local, but that may be facilitated by sedoanalgesia in the operating room. However, patients have expectations for rapid discharge home with a level of functionality similar to that associated with an office visit. The use of longer-acting sedatives or opioids is unwarranted.

Topicalization of the airway is accomplished as described earlier. Supplemental oxygen and capnometry are instituted via nasal cannula and ondansetron (4 mg) given intravenously. Remifentanil is the optimal opioid for these procedures. A bolus (0.2–0.5 μg/kg) is administered immediately before scope insertion followed by infusion at 0.05 to 0.15 μg/kg/min. The remifentanil infusion can be titrated to respiratory rate and patient comfort. Within minutes of procedure completion patients are essentially fully recovered and ready for fast-track discharge.

A modified anesthetic technique allows diagnostic upper aerodigestive tract procedures to be performed in an expedient, comfortable manner with minimum morbidity.[71] Because patients are breathing spontaneously they are able to attempt phonation, cough, and swallow on command, allowing the surgeon to assess movement of the vocal folds and tracheomalacia. If needed, biopsies can also be performed easily.

Esophagoscopy (Both Transnasal and Per Oral Esophagoscopy)

This procedure can be performed comfortably with mild sedation and topical nasal anesthesia and decongestion.[72] Esophagoscopy is indicated as a diagnostic tool for patients with dysphagia, in cancer surveillance, and for patients with reflux. Biopsies or esophageal dilation of a stricture can also be performed with ease. The transnasal or oral approaches can be used. If the transnasal route is undertaken then nasal decongestion is critical. Because the patients are awake, they in fact assist by swallowing air along with air insufflation. This procedure can be done in the office or endoscopy suite, and the comfort afforded by the anesthetic remifentanil has made this much more tolerable for the patient. Moreover, if dilation is performed a small mucosal tear is commonly created. Spontaneous ventilation, as opposed to positive pressure mask, may also serve to decrease the risk of iatrogenic dissection or expansion of the tear.

Laryngeal Stenosis

Determination of the level and extent is critical in the management of these conditions. Awake laryngoscopy and bronchoscopy under topical anesthesia with intravenous remifentanil as described earlier (small bolus + titrated infusion) is ideal for this evaluation. The procedure is safe, as patients are breathing spontaneously, and also allows assessment of the dynamics of the airway including vocal fold mobility and airway collapsibility. Unlike in the office, a decision to perform an immediate intervention can also be made. Examples would include balloon dilatation or even tracheostomy. If the latter is to be undertaken, the operating suite provides a controlled environment with skilled perioperative support whereby such surgery can be immediately performed. For a balloon dilatation, the dilator is generally passed through the nose parallel to the flexible endoscope and allows visualization of the dilatation process under a safer setting.[73] Similarly, tracheal dilation often produces a clinically insignificant mucosal tear. Positive pressure ventilation during general anesthesia with endotracheal intubation may present a risk of expansion and gas embolus.

Laser Endoscopy of Larynx and Trachea

Some patients will be scheduled for therapeutic ablation of a laryngeal lesion, often with laser using the flexible fiberoptic technique.[74] Patient immobility or full cooperation during critical periods and analgesia are important elements of the anesthetic. Remifentanil infusion with topical anesthesia is often adequate. General anesthesia with an LMA (see the article by Jeff E. Mandel elsewhere in this issue) is one option. Sedation with DEX-ketamine as described for thyroplasty is another option, while laser surgery with local anesthesia and no sedation has been advocated by others.[75] Patient-specific factors and surgeon experience will certainly be significant factors in determining a suitable anesthetic approach.

Controlled analgesia and anesthesia along with the application of local anesthetics can permit laryngeal laser procedures without the placement of large laser endotracheal tubes, which make visualization of glottic, subglottic, and upper tracheal lesions challenging. Patients are breathing spontaneously and flexible lasers, both CO_2 and KTP, can be used depending on the specific pathology of the lesions. For papilloma and vascular lesions such as ecstatic capillaries, granulomas, and hemorrhagic spots, chromophore-directed lasers like the KTP laser are efficacious.[76] Fiber lasers can be passed through a bronchoscope and an aiming beam is desirable. Biopsies may be performed prior to vaporization of lesions. Drawbacks to this procedure include the constant movement of the vocal folds with respiration, and pain, which is however well controlled with the analgesia provided. Because there is limited need for high inspired oxygen concentrations in most spontaneously breathing patients, the risk of airway fires is much less but safety goggles and wet drapes are necessary. In addition, laser system maintenance is easier in endoscopy suites.

Vocal Fold Injections for Medialization

These procedures are often performed for a recent-onset vocal fold paralysis whereby a patient presents with breathy dysphonia and aspiration.[77,78] Other indications include age-related vocal fold atrophy. The procedure can be performed through several approaches, including transcartilaginous, through the cricothyroid or thyrohyoid membranes, or orally. The patient's ability to phonate on command during the procedure is a definite advantage, and mild coughing can help disperse the injectable along the vocal fold more evenly. The medications administered help allay patient anxiety and suppress the cough reflexes. Drawbacks to an awake approach include movement of the vocal folds during respiration and inadequate visualization, especially if the patient is experiencing discomfort, and improper placement of the injectable into the submucosa. The addition of low-dose intravenous analgesia or titratable sedation mitigates these problems. All these injections are performed with the patient awake, breathing spontaneously, and able to phonate on command.

As with biopsies and laser procedures, a minimal amount of bleeding at the site may be encountered. Spraying Afrin (oxymetazoline) through the side port of a bronchoscope or laryngoscope will effect hemostasis. Botulinum toxin can also be injected in to the thyroarytenoideus by the same technique.

Tracheoesophageal Puncture

A tracheoesophageal puncture is a surgical procedure performed to rehabilitate the voice in a patient who has undergone a total laryngectomy.[72] The procedure involves creation of a fistula between the trachea and the esophagus. A prosthesis or a red rubber catheter is then placed through this fistula. If a catheter is placed it is then replaced by a prosthesis after approximately 1 week. The prosthesis is a one-way valve that keeps food out of the trachea but lets air into the esophagus for esophageal speech. A tracheoesophageal puncture can be performed with the help of a transnasal or small-caliber esophagoscope. The procedure involves air insufflation through an esophagoscope at the esophageal inlet while a second surgeon creates the puncture and fistula through the tracheostoma. The main risk is coughing and aspiration of blood during the procedure. Coughing is controlled by topicalization or low-dose sedoanalgesia.[79]

Gore-Tex Medialization Thyroplasty

The indications for a permanent treatment of unilateral vocal fold paralysis (UVFP) are usually the resultant dysphonia, ineffective cough, and aspiration in a patient with either a long-standing vocal fold paralysis or one in whom the nerve has been deliberately resected, as in the treatment of a thyroid cancer. Laryngeal framework surgery is the gold standard for the treatment of UVFP. The concept of medialization thyroplasty is to medialize the paralyzed vocal fold from an external approach and work through the thyroid cartilage. A small window is created at the mid level of the thyroid cartilage and an implant of Gore-Tex, Silastic, or a commercially available material is placed through the window to medialize the paralyzed vocal fold. Voice quality is monitored intraoperatively both perceptually and with laryngeal examination via flexible laryngoscopy. Such monitoring allows the surgeon to adjust the surgery to optimize the voice quality and improve maximum phonation time at the end of the procedure, which is a critical element to this surgery and is best performed under monitored anesthesia without intubation and general anesthesia.

Thyroplasty is usually performed on an extended-stay outpatient basis (ie, overnight observation). Potential short-term complications include vocal fold or surgical site hemorrhage, implant displacement/extrusion, and acute airway obstruction.

Medialization thyroplasty can be performed under general anesthesia with an LMA while visualizing the vocal cords endoscopically through the LMA.[80] LMA use for these, and related ear/nose/throat procedures, is reviewed in the article by Jeff E. Mandel elsewhere in this issue. General anesthesia with an LMA using an asleep-awake-asleep approach has also been described. Thyroplasty performed under general anesthesia may be preceded by a separate office procedure involving collagen injection to help determine the cord position associated with optimal voice improvement.[81] This approach is less practical and a less efficient use of resources. When general endotracheal intubation is performed for collagen injection, the local trauma of the tube may actually compress the injected region thereby reducing efficacy of the injection. The displacement of a thyroplasty implant during subsequent intubation has also been reported.[82]

Surgeons generally agree that sedation with periodic intraoperative assessment of patient phonation is the optimal approach. Advantages of sedation include intraoperative vocalization for real-time voice assessment of graft placement, and decreased risk of further vocal cord/nerve injury related to airway instrumentation. When performed under sedation, deep sedation is avoided and moderate "cooperative" sedation is planned. A less optimal approach requires reversal of benzodiazepine-induced deep sedation with flumazenil to facilitate voice assessment.[83] The balance between adequate sedation and cooperation can be difficult to achieve and is very unpredictable with standard combinations of benzodiazepines and opioids. DEX offers an alternative approach with promising early results.[84]

The combination of DEX with ketamine is an evolving approach for Gore-Tex medialization thyroplasty and is the standard approach at the authors' institution. Airway topicalization is not necessary, but nasal block with lidocaine and topical vasoconstrictor are beneficial for the diagnostic component. DEX load (1 μg/kg over 10 min) is usually started immediately on patient transfer to the operating table. If midazolam is used, the initial dose (0.5–1 mg) is given at this time. The optimal sedation end point is maintained, spontaneous eye closure by the patient who is still arousable to stimulus but does not spontaneously self-arouse. If this state is achieved before completion of the DEX load, the bolus can be aborted and infusion (0.5 μg/kg/h) started and adjusted to appropriate maintenance (0.1–1 μg/kg/h). Nasopharyngeal laryngoscopy to assess vocal cord movement during patient phonation is performed at the outset, before skin preparation, and intraoperatively to assess function during positioning of the implant through the thyroid window. In some cases transnasal visualization of the glottic opening can be challenging because of soft tissue overlap. Placement of a 28F nasal trumpet lubricated with lidocaine can facilitate the nasopharyngeal laryngoscopic examination. The airway can be left in place for subsequent examination. Capnometry is instituted via nasal cannula, and supplemental oxygen can be delivered as needed. Oxygen flow can be reduced or turned off during the use of electrocautery. A ketamine bolus (0.25–0.5 mg/kg) is administered shortly before injection of local anesthetic by the surgeon. Ketamine infusion (3–10 μg/kg/min) can be instituted at this time or alternatively reserved to supplement the anesthetic later, if necessary. For patients in whom ketamine is deemed contraindicated, a remifentanil infusion (0.05–0.1 μg/kg/min) without bolus can be initiated during the DEX load to provide analgesia for local injection.

CASE SCENARIO

A 55-year-old woman (height 165 cm, weight 185 kg) presented to the office of the laryngologist with a vocal fold paralysis. She had previously undergone a total thyroidectomy and neck dissection for aggressive medullary thyroid cancer. In fact her cancer was diagnosed as part of the workup for her sudden onset of hoarseness, and she had a vocal fold paralysis prior to her surgery. At the time of her surgery her surgeon found the recurrent laryngeal nerve to be grossly involved with the cancer, and the nerve was resected. At the time of her presentation she complained of breathy dysphonia, aspiration with oral liquid consumption, and an ineffective cough. She was scheduled for radiation, and wanted her voice and swallowing addressed before this treatment commenced.

She had no other significant medical history including any negative history of sleep apnea or snoring. Examination revealed a Class II airway with no other predictors of a difficult airway. She was counseled on the benefits of performing the procedure under sedation with the need for intraoperative participation (phonation) and the likelihood of recall of the procedure.

She was brought to the operating room, where 1 mg of midazolam and 4 mg of ondansetron were administered and American Society of Anesthesiologists standard monitors placed. The patient self-administered oxymetazoline spray to the nares. A DEX load (1 μg/kg over 10 min) was initiated via an intravenous line attached to the catheter hub to a pigtail adapter and a check-valve intravenous microdrip. Both arms were tucked at the sides and padded. The right naris was anesthetized by placement of 3 cotton-tipped applicators soaked in 4% lidocaine. Seven minutes into the DEX load the patient was asleep but arousable, demonstrating maintained spontaneous eye closure and minimal response to manipulation of the nasal applicators. The load was stopped and a continuous infusion at 0.5 μg/kg/h started. An examination of the vocal cords during patient phonation was performed via a transnasal fiberoptic scope. A nasal cannula with continuous oral capnometry was placed and 2 L/min oxygen flow initiated. The patient was bolused 40 mg of ketamine (1%), and with the onset of nystagmus 10 mL of 1% lidocaine with 1:200,000 epinephrine local anesthetic was placed by the surgeon at the incision site. A ketamine infusion was initiated at 5 μg/kg/min. The head was covered with a plastic face shield that was covered with sterile drapes and towels. She underwent a unilateral Gore-Tex thyroplasty through the thyroidectomy incision. The Gore-Tex graft was placed via a window created in the thyroid cartilage. A transnasal fiberoptic examination of the vocal cords was performed by the surgical assistant to assess voice and glottic closure as the optimal graft position was determined. The graft was sutured in place and the incision closed. Total operating time was 125 minutes. The patient remained cooperative and responsive to command throughout. Good glottic closure was obtained as well as an immediate improvement in her voice and swallowing at the end of the procedure, at which time infusions were stopped. In the PACU the patient was comfortable and required intermittent fentanyl (25 μg) for moderate discomfort. Her blood pressure and heart rate remained 10% to 20% below baseline for the first hour. She stated that she recalled parts of the surgery but generally felt comfortable, albeit while experiencing a strange feeling that she was "involved in a cartoon." She was admitted for overnight airway observation, the drain was removed in the morning, and she was discharged home the next day.

SUMMARY

The range of surgical procedures for treatment of laryngeal pathology continues to broaden. Such procedures are increasingly performed in the ambulatory surgery-based or office-based setting under local anesthesia with controlled, cooperative sedation. A thorough appreciation of the pharmacodynamic interactions and pharmacokinetics of commonly used sedation agents is crucial to safe and expeditious sedation for airway surgery. DEX and combinations of DEX with low doses of sedative adjuncts is a promising anesthetic approach for subtypes of "awake" airway surgery, especially thyroplasty and tracheostomy. Collaboration with the surgeon and setting appropriate patient expectations in perioperative anesthetic management and planning will facilitate success. Patients who are otherwise reluctant to be treated in the office-based setting can get access to important diagnostic and therapeutic interventions in the safety of the operating room setting without the recovery profile and attendant morbidities of general anesthesia.

REFERENCES

1. Hutchinson RC, Kenny GN. Sedation for endoscopy. Curr Opin Anaesthesiol 2000;13(4):415–9.
2. Macchiarini P, Rovira I, Ferrarello S. Awake upper airway surgery. Ann Thorac Surg 2010;89(2):387–90 [discussion 390–1].
3. Benumof JL, editor. Airway management: principles and practice. St. Louis (MO): C. V. Mosby; 1996.
4. Finlay WH, Martin AR. Recent advances in predictive understanding of respiratory tract deposition. J Aerosol Med Pulm Drug Deliv 2008;21(2):189–206.
5. Woodruff C, Wieczorek PM, Schricker T, et al. Atomised lidocaine for airway topical anaesthesia in the morbidly obese: 1% compared with 2%. Anaesthesia 2010;65(1):12–7.
6. Wieczorek PM, Schricker T, Vinet B, et al. Airway topicalisation in morbidly obese patients using atomised lidocaine: 2% compared with 4%. Anaesthesia 2007; 62(10):984–8.
7. Tsui BC, Cunningham K. Fiberoptic endotracheal intubation after topicalization with in-circuit nebulized lidocaine in a child with a difficult airway. Anesth Analg 2004;98(5):1286–8.
8. Isaac PA, Barry JE, Vaughan RS, et al. A jet nebuliser for delivery of topical anesthesia to the respiratory tract. A comparison with cricothyroid puncture and direct spraying for fibreoptic bronchoscopy. Anaesthesia 1990;45(1):46–8.

9. Kirkpatrick MB, Sanders RV, Bass JB Jr. Physiologic effects and serum lidocaine concentrations after inhalation of lidocaine from a compressed gas-powered jet nebulizer. Am Rev Respir Dis 1987;136(2):447–9.

10. Weinberg GL. Limits to lipid in the literature and lab: what we know, what we don't know. Anesth Analg 2009;108(4):1062–4.

11. Berger R, McConnell JW, Phillips B, et al. Safety and efficacy of using high-dose topical and nebulized anesthesia to obtain endobronchial cultures. Chest 1989; 95(2):299–303.

12. Bhattacharyya N, Gopal HV. Examining the safety of nasogastric tube placement after endoscopic sinus surgery. Ann Otol Rhinol Laryngol 1998;107(8):662–4.

13. Greenland KB, Irwin MG. The Williams Airway Intubator, the Ovassapian Airway and the Berman Airway as upper airway conduits for fibreoptic bronchoscopy in patients with difficult airways. Curr Opin Anaesthesiol 2004;17(6):505–10.

14. Canning BJ, Chou YL. Cough sensors. I. Physiological and pharmacological properties of the afferent nerves regulating cough. Handb Exp Pharmacol 2009;187:23–47.

15. Guler G, Akin A, Tosun Z, et al. Single-dose dexmedetomidine attenuates airway and circulatory reflexes during extubation. Acta Anaesthesiol Scand 2005;49(8): 1088–91.

16. Undem BJ, Carr MJ. Targeting primary afferent nerves for novel antitussive therapy. Chest 2010;137(1):177–84.

17. Pattinson KT, Governo RJ, MacIntosh BJ, et al. Opioids depress cortical centers responsible for the volitional control of respiration. J Neurosci 2009;29(25):8177–86.

18. Machata AM, Illievich UM, Gustorff B, et al. Remifentanil for tracheal tube tolerance: a case control study. Anaesthesia 2007;62(8):796–801.

19. Gustorff B, Felleiter P, Nahlik G, et al. The effect of remifentanil on the heat pain threshold in volunteers. Anesth Analg 2001;92(2):369–74.

20. Xu YC, Xue FS, Luo MP, et al. Median effective dose of remifentanil for awake laryngoscopy and intubation. Chin Med J (Engl) 2009;122(13):1507–12.

21. Fu ES, Downs JB, Schweiger JW, et al. Supplemental oxygen impairs detection of hypoventilation by pulse oximetry. Chest 2004;126(5):1552–8.

22. Bernards CM, Knowlton SL, Schmidt DF, et al. Respiratory and sleep effects of remifentanil in volunteers with moderate obstructive sleep apnea. Anesthesiology 2009;110(1):41–9.

23. Egan TD, Huizinga B, Gupta SK, et al. Remifentanil pharmacokinetics in obese versus lean patients. Anesthesiology 1998;89(3):562–73.

24. Hay JL, White JM, Bochner F, et al. Antinociceptive effects of high dose remifentanil in male methadone-maintained patients. Eur J Pain 2008;12:926–33.

25. Apfel CC, Bacher A, Biedler A, et al. A factorial trial of six interventions for the prevention of postoperative nausea and vomiting. Anaesthesist 2005;54(3):201–9.

26. Dershwitz M, Michalowski P, Chang Y, et al. Postoperative nausea and vomiting after total intravenous anesthesia with propofol and remifentanil or alfentanil: how important is the opioid? J Clin Anesth 2002;14(4):275–8.

27. Song D, Whitten CW, White PF. Remifentanil infusion facilitates early recovery for obese outpatients undergoing laparoscopic cholecystectomy. Anesth Analg 2000;90(5):1111–3.

28. Avramov MN, Smith I, White PF. Interactions between midazolam and remifentanil during monitored anesthesia care. Anesthesiology 1996;85(6):1283–9.

29. Gold MI, Watkins WD, Sung YF, et al. Remifentanil versus remifentanil/midazolam for ambulatory surgery during monitored anesthesia care. Anesthesiology 1997; 87(1):51–7.

30. Kilpatrick GJ, McIntyre MS, Cox RF, et al. CNS 7056: a novel ultra-short-acting benzodiazepine. Anesthesiology 2007;107(1):60–6.
31. Williams TJ, Bowie PE. Midazolam sedation to produce complete amnesia for bronchoscopy: 2 years' experience at a district general hospital. Respir Med 1999;93(5):361–5.
32. Clark G, Licker M, Younossian AB, et al. Titrated sedation with propofol or midazolam for flexible bronchoscopy: a randomised trial. Eur Respir J 2009;34(6): 1277–83.
33. Hendrickx JF, Eger EI 2nd, Sonner JM, et al. Is synergy the rule? A review of anesthetic interactions producing hypnosis and immobility. Anesth Analg 2008;107(2): 494–506.
34. Bailey PL, Pace NL, Ashburn MA, et al. Frequent hypoxemia and apnea after sedation with midazolam and fentanyl. Anesthesiology 1990;73(5):826–30.
35. Litman RS, McDonough JM, Marcus CL, et al. Upper airway collapsibility in anesthetized children. Anesth Analg 2006;102(3):750–4.
36. Drummond GB. Comparison of sedation with midazolam and ketamine: effects on airway muscle activity. Br J Anaesth 1996;76(5):663–7.
37. Litman RS. Upper airway collapsibility: an emerging paradigm for measuring the safety of anesthetic and sedative agents. Anesthesiology 2005;103(3):453–4.
38. Ikeda H, Ayuse T, Oi K. The effects of head and body positioning on upper airway collapsibility in normal subjects who received midazolam sedation. J Clin Anesth 2006;18(3):185–93.
39. Ben-Shlomo I, Tverskoy M, Fleyshman G, et al. Intramuscular administration of lidocaine or bupivacaine alters the effect of midazolam from sedation to hypnosis in a dose-dependent manner. J Basic Clin Physiol Pharmacol 2003;14(3):257–63.
40. Lichtenbelt BJ, Olofsen E, Dahan A, et al. Propofol reduces the distribution and clearance of midazolam. Anesth Analg 2010;110:1597–606.
41. Negus BH, Street NE. Midazolam-opioid combination and postoperative upper airway obstruction in children. Anaesth Intensive Care 1994;22(2):232–3.
42. Tian SY, Zou L, Quan X, et al. Effect of midazolam on memory: a study of process dissociation procedure and functional magnetic resonance imaging. Anaesthesia 2010;65:586–94.
43. Shukry M, Miller JA. Update on dexmedetomidine: use in nonintubated patients requiring sedation for surgical procedures. Ther Clin Risk Manag 2010;6:111–21.
44. Huncke T, Chan J, Doyle W, et al. The use of continuous positive airway pressure during an awake craniotomy in a patient with obstructive sleep apnea. J Clin Anesth 2008;20(4):297–9.
45. Candiotti KA, Bergese SD, Bokesch PM, et al. Monitored anesthesia care with dexmedetomidine: a prospective, randomized, double-blind, multicenter trial. Anesth Analg 2010;110(1):47–56.
46. Hsu YW, Cortinez LI, Robertson KM, et al. Dexmedetomidine pharmacodynamics: part I: crossover comparison of the respiratory effects of dexmedetomidine and remifentanil in healthy volunteers. Anesthesiology 2004;101(5):1066–76.
47. Mahmoud M, Radhakrishnan R, Gunter J, et al. Effect of increasing depth of dexmedetomidine anesthesia on upper airway morphology in children. Paediatr Anaesth 2010;20:506–15.
48. van Oostrom H, Stienen PJ, Doornenbal A, et al. The alpha(2)-adrenoceptor agonist dexmedetomidine suppresses memory formation only at doses attenuating the perception of sensory input. Eur J Pharmacol 2010;629(1–3):58–62.
49. Ustun Y, Gunduz M, Erdogan O, et al. Dexmedetomidine versus midazolam in outpatient third molar surgery. J Oral Maxillofac Surg 2006;64(9):1353–8.

50. Bergese SD, Patrick Bender S, McSweeney TD, et al. A comparative study of dexmedetomidine with midazolam and midazolam alone for sedation during elective awake fiberoptic intubation. J Clin Anesth 2010;22(1):35–40.
51. Gilsbach R, Roser C, Beetz N, et al. Genetic dissection of alpha2-adrenoceptor functions in adrenergic versus nonadrenergic cells. Mol Pharmacol 2009;75(5):1160–70.
52. Arcangeli A, D'Alo C, Gaspari R. Dexmedetomidine use in general anaesthesia. Curr Drug Targets 2009;10(8):687–95.
53. Bailey PL, Sperry RJ, Johnson GK, et al. Respiratory effects of clonidine alone and combined with morphine, in humans. Anesthesiology 1991;74(1):43–8.
54. Haenggi M, Ypparila-Wolters H, Hauser K, et al. Intra- and inter-individual variation of BIS-index(R) and Entropy(R) during controlled sedation with midazolam/remifentanil and dexmedetomidine/remifentanil in healthy volunteers: an interventional study. Crit Care 2009;13(1):R20.
55. Busick T, Kussman M, Scheidt T, et al. Preliminary experience with dexmedetomidine for monitored anesthesia care during ENT surgical procedures. Am J Ther 2008;15(6):520–7.
56. Mankikian B, Cantineau JP, Sartene R, et al. Ventilatory pattern and chest wall mechanics during ketamine anesthesia in humans. Anesthesiology 1986;65(5):492–9.
57. Persson J, Scheinin H, Hellstrom G, et al. Ketamine antagonises alfentanil-induced hypoventilation in healthy male volunteers. Acta Anaesthesiol Scand 1999;43(7):744–52.
58. Levanen J, Makela ML, Scheinin H. Dexmedetomidine premedication attenuates ketamine-induced cardiostimulatory effects and postanesthetic delirium. Anesthesiology 1995;82(5):1117–25.
59. Remerand F, Le Tendre C, Baud A, et al. The early and delayed analgesic effects of ketamine after total hip arthroplasty: a prospective, randomized, controlled, double-blind study. Anesth Analg 2009;109(6):1963–71.
60. Wathen JE, Roback MG, Mackenzie T, et al. Does midazolam alter the clinical effects of intravenous ketamine sedation in children? A double-blind, randomized, controlled, emergency department trial. Ann Emerg Med 2000;36(6):579–88.
61. Subramaniam K, Subramaniam B, Steinbrook RA. Ketamine as adjuvant analgesic to opioids: a quantitative and qualitative systematic review. Anesth Analg 2004;99(2):482–95, table of contents.
62. Iravani M, Wald SH. Dexmedetomidine and ketamine for fiberoptic intubation in a child with severe mandibular hypoplasia. J Clin Anesth 2008;20(6):455–7.
63. Mester R, Easley RB, Brady KM, et al. Monitored anesthesia care with a combination of ketamine and dexmedetomidine during cardiac catheterization. Am J Ther 2008;15(1):24–30.
64. Mahmoud M, Tyler T, Sadhasivam S. Dexmedetomidine and ketamine for large anterior mediastinal mass biopsy. Paediatr Anaesth 2008;18(10):1011–3.
65. Scher CS, Gitlin MC. Dexmedetomidine and low-dose ketamine provide adequate sedation for awake fibreoptic intubation. Can J Anaesth 2003;50(6):607–10.
66. Rosen CA, Amin MR, Sulica L, et al. Advances in office-based diagnosis and treatment in laryngology. Laryngoscope 2009;119(Suppl 2):S185–212.
67. Bastian RW, Delsupehe KG. Indirect larynx and pharynx surgery: a replacement for direct laryngoscopy. Laryngoscope 1996;106(10):1280–6.
68. Eller R, Ginsburg M, Lurie D, et al. Flexible laryngoscopy: a comparison of fiber optic and distal chip technologies—part 2: laryngopharyngeal reflux. J Voice 2009;23(3):389–95.

69. Eller R, Ginsburg M, Lurie D, et al. Flexible laryngoscopy: a comparison of fiber optic and distal chip technologies. Part 1: vocal fold masses. J Voice 2008;22(6): 746–50.

70. Postma GN, Amin MR, Simpson CB, et al. Office procedures for the esophagus. Ear Nose Throat J 2004;83(7 Suppl 2):17–21.

71. Sulica L, Blitzer A. Anesthesia for laryngeal surgery in the office. Laryngoscope 2000;110(10 Pt 1):1777–9.

72. Bach KK, Postma GN, Koufman JA. In-office tracheoesophageal puncture using transnasal esophagoscopy. Laryngoscope 2003;113(1):173–6.

73. Lee KH, Rutter MJ. Role of balloon dilation in the management of adult idiopathic subglottic stenosis. Ann Otol Rhinol Laryngol 2008;117(2):81–4.

74. Ossoff RH, Coleman JA, Courey MS, et al. Clinical applications of lasers in otolaryngology—head and neck surgery. Lasers Surg Med 1994;15(3):217–48.

75. Zeitels SM, Burns JA. Office-based laryngeal laser surgery with local anesthesia. Curr Opin Otolaryngol Head Neck Surg 2007;15(3):141–7.

76. McMillan K, Shapshay SM, McGilligan JA, et al. A 585-nanometer pulsed dye laser treatment of laryngeal papillomas: preliminary report. Laryngoscope 1998;108(7):968–72.

77. Bogdasarian RS, Olson NR. Posterior glottic laryngeal stenosis. Otolaryngol Head Neck Surg 1980;88(6):765–72.

78. Sulica L, Blitzer A. Vocal fold paresis: evidence and controversies. Curr Opin Otolaryngol Head Neck Surg 2007;15(3):159–62.

79. Johns ME, Cantrell RW. Voice restoration of the total laryngectomy patient: the Singer-Blom technique. Otolaryngol Head Neck Surg 1981;89(1):82–6.

80. Razzaq I, Wooldridge W. A series of thyroplasty cases under general anaesthesia. Br J Anaesth 2000;85(4):547–9.

81. Sproson E, Nightingale J, Puxeddu R. Thyroplasty type I under general anaesthesia with the use of the laryngeal mask and a waking period to assess voice. Auris Nasus Larynx 2010;37(3):357–60.

82. Ayala MA, Patterson MB, Bach KK. Late displacement of a Montgomery thyroplasty implant following endotracheal intubation. Ann Otol Rhinol Laryngol 2007;116(4):262–4.

83. Donnelly M, Browne J, Fitzpatrick G. Anaesthesia for thyroplasty. Can J Anaesth 1995;42(9):813–5.

84. Jense RJ, Souter K, Davies J, et al. Dexmedetomidine sedation for laryngeal framework surgery. Ann Otol Rhinol Laryngol 2008;117(9):659–64.

Index

Note: Page numbers of article titles are in **boldface** type.

Moving?

Make sure your subscription moves with you!

To notify us of your new address, find your **Clinics Account Number** (located on your mailing label above your name), and contact customer service at:

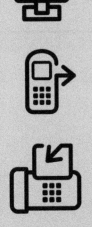

Email: journalscustomerservice-usa@elsevier.com

800-654-2452 (subscribers in the U.S. & Canada)
314-447-8871 (subscribers outside of the U.S. & Canada)

Fax number: 314-447-8029

Elsevier Health Sciences Division
Subscription Customer Service
3251 Riverport Lane
Maryland Heights, MO 63043

*To ensure uninterrupted delivery of your subscription, please notify us at least 4 weeks in advance of move.

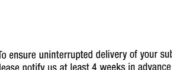
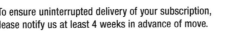

Printed and bound by CPI Group (UK) Ltd, Croydon, CR0 4YY

03/10/2024

01040453-0020